MEDICAL WRITING
The Technic and the Art

MEDICAL WRITING
The Technic and the Art

FOURTH EDITION

By

MORRIS FISHBEIN, M.D.

Editor, Medical World News
New York, New York
Medical Editor, Britannica Book of the Year
Formerly Editor, The Journal of the American Medical Association

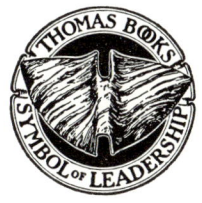

CHARLES C THOMAS • PUBLISHER
Springfield • Illinois • U.S.A.

Published and Distributed Throughout the World by
CHARLES C THOMAS • PUBLISHER
BANNERSTONE HOUSE
301-327 East Lawrence Avenue, Springfield, Illinois, U.S.A.
NATCHEZ PLANTATION HOUSE
735 North Atlantic Boulevard, Fort Lauderdale, Florida, U.S.A.

This book is protected by copyright. No part of it may be reproduced in any manner without written permission from the publisher.

© *1938, 1948, and 1957, by* McGraw-Hill Book Company Inc.
© *1972, by* CHARLES C THOMAS • PUBLISHER
Standard Book Number: 398-02279-8
Library of Congress Catalog Card Number 73-165883

First Edition, 1938
Second Edition, 1948
Third Edition, 1957
Fourth Edition, 1972

With THOMAS BOOKS *careful attention is given to all details of manufacturing and design. It is the Publisher's desire to present books that are satisfactory as to their physical qualities and artistic possibilities and appropriate for their particular use.* THOMAS BOOKS *will be true to those laws of quality that assure a good name and good will.*

Printed in the United States of America
N-10

PREFACE

THIS BOOK REPRESENTS the evolution of theory and practice on medical writing in my association with the editorial department of the American Medical Association for some thirty-five years and more recently with *Medical World News, Excerpta Medica* and other publications. When Dr. George H. Simmons became editor of *The Journal of the American Medical Association* he accumulated various memorandums concerned with the preparation of papers for publication. Later I assisted him in preparing an essay entitled "Art and Practice of Medical Writing." The present volume constitutes an extensive revision of previous editions together with much new material.

The help of the following persons, whose suggestions are incorporated in this book, is acknowledged with appreciation: Marjorie Hutchins Moore, for many years librarian of the American Medical Association; F. K. Bryant; Dr. Austin Smith; and Dr. Howard Fox, late editor emeritus of the *Archives of Dermatology and Syphilology*, who assisted in the preparation of the section on Latin and Greek terminology.

The late Jewel F. Whelan, my assistant for more than twenty years, aided greatly in assembling material for this book. She had a veritable passion for accuracy and the meticulous editing of scientific papers.

Grateful acknowledgment is made also to William Brown McNett for material included in the chapter on illustrations and for the preparation of several illustrations, and to Laura E. Moore for the chapter on indexing.

MORRIS FISHBEIN, M.D.

INTRODUCTION

THE QUALITY of contributions to medical literature is constantly improving. Far too often, however, physicians still prepare their contributions with a striving and agony and delay comparable to the delivery of human progeny by one untutored in the refinements of obstetrics. Often the physician who is asked to prepare for a medical society a review of available knowledge on a subject fails to inform himself of the innumerable agencies prepared to assist him in accomplishing what should be a simple task. He is likely to seat himself in his office or in his den at home, surround himself with a liberal quantity of textbooks and periodicals selected at random and then endeavor to collate this material in a single evening. What the physician fails to realize is the importance of preparing a systematic, orderly, scientific outline as the first step in writing on any subject. He overlooks the significance of having an introduction, a body, a summary and a conclusion in any type of scientific essay.

Professional writers in every field of literature realize the importance of preparing a manuscript for the publication for which it is meant. Some periodicals limit themselves to articles of 1,500 words; others are capable of handling large monographic presentations. *The Journal of the American Medical Association,* for instance, endeavors to limit practically all scientific contributions to six pages, or not more than 6,000 words (preferably less). When articles are prepared for a specific purpose, greater latitude may be granted. Obviously the physician who is preparing an article for a state medical journal, for one of the periodicals devoted to a medical specialty or for any other medical periodical should be familiar with the nature of the publication and should plan his article according to the usual pattern followed by that publication.

Many a medical writer has said that such limitations interfere seriously with proper display of his individuality. Actually, a writer may utilize his literary accomplishments and style to better advantage under some such orderly plan than when he gives free rein to his imagination and writes as the spirit moves him. One of my most respected teachers once said that the outward appearance of a manuscript, its arrangement, the quality of its spelling and punctuation and its choice of diction were excellent indications of the personal characteristics and scientific qualifications of the writer. The clinician or the research worker in the laboratory betrays in his literary contributions the possession of a scientific mind or the lack of it.

Competition is certainly as great in medical writing as in medical practice. The leading medical publications are overwhelmed with offers of material. Many of the periodicals devoted to medical specialties find it necessary to hold manuscripts from six months to a year or more before space can be found for their publication. Therefore, the physician who launches a literary venture poorly clad, unsound in its constitution, limping in some of its sections and bruised by bad grammar may expect to have his manuscript returned with the statement, "The editor regrets...."

The National Association of Science Writers, Inc., has issued a guide to free-lance writers which is helpful in determining how to prepare manuscripts and get them published. If the physician, or any other writer, develops an idea for an article, he may first assemble in outline form his idea of what the article should contain, as well as the necessary bibliographic references on which the article will be based. He may then select a suitable periodical editor or agent who he thinks may be interested in publishing such an article. He should not submit his idea at the same time to several editors or publications. He should choose in order those which he thinks might be interested and then address one after another. If the editor or the agency wishes to have the writer complete the article or a series of articles or a book, he will respond by informing the writer. Such a letter may tell the author when the article must be completed, the length of the manuscript, any ideas which the editor feels might be covered and other important information. He may also propose a fee which will be paid at the completion of the agreement (known as an advance) and also the

Introduction

fee to be paid when the article or book is delivered. He may send a contract which will supply all of the necessary information about the details of the agreement under which the writer works.

In preparing an article or a book, the writer will already have assembled enough material to indicate the lines to be followed. However, he will need additional data. Any quotations should be verified and properly indicated bibliographically. In many instances a release by the owner of the copyright will be necessary in order to reproduce the quotation.

After an article is written, the writer may wish to study it to make sure that he has met the requirements of the editor or agency for whom the material has been prepared. If this has not been done or if new material has been added of which the editor or agency has not had notice, the writer should inform the editor immediately of what has been done. He may then modify the article or even expand certain areas in accordance with the wishes of the editor.

A deadline is the final date at which the editor or agency expects to receive the article, the manuscript or whatever material has been prepared. Editors are not too much disturbed if an article is received well before the time of the deadline. Since, however, they may have made plans for the use of the material, most editors or publishers will not tolerate unwarranted delay in meeting the deadline.

When an editor or a publisher accepts a manuscript he may or may not inform the author as to the expected date when it will be published. If the author is anxious, he may inquire as to the date of publication. Often, however, editors or publishers are unable to supply such information. Manuscripts may be held for varying periods of time before it is possible to include them in a periodical or to publish a book as a part of the season's output. Some editors will hesitate to make their own decisions after receiving a manuscript. They may wish to send it to a reviewer or several reviewers who will be asked to give opinions. If there are doubts, the manuscript may be held for a considerable time before publication. The reviewers may suggest omissions, additions or changes which the editor may wish to submit to the writer for his final decision.

CONTENTS

	Page
Preface	v
Introduction	vii

Chapter

1.	An Acceptable Paper	3
2.	Style	8
3.	The Subject and the Material	26
4.	Construction of the Manuscript	39
5.	Words and Phrases	46
6.	Spelling	83
7.	Capitalization	106
8.	Abbreviations	108
9.	Numbers	118
10.	Pharmaceutic Products and Prescriptions	127
11.	Bibliographic Material	131
12.	Preparation of the Manuscript	143
13.	Illustrations	149
14.	Tables and Charts	165
15.	Revision of the Manuscript	176
16.	Proofreading	182
17.	Indexing	187

Index 195

MEDICAL WRITING
The Technic and the Art

1
AN ACCEPTABLE PAPER

THE WRITING and publication of articles are significant in the development of a successful physician. By these he becomes known outside his own community. Through the reading of papers before societies, he makes himself and his work known to hundreds; through his publications, to thousands. Even more important, the writing of an article helps to make the writer better informed on the subject he discusses.

CAUSES FOR THE REJECTION OF MANUSCRIPTS

The majority of the manuscripts voluntarily offered to leading medical publications are returned. What are the reasons for their rejection?

Lack of Space

The great number of medical organizations that hold meetings produce thousands of papers which are usually submitted for publication. Lack of space is a primary cause for rejection. But no matter how many papers the periodical may have on hand, a well-prepared article which will appeal to a large proportion of readers —especially to general practitioners—is usually accepted. Indeed a wise editor will promptly accept a manuscript that offers new material and publish it ahead of others less significant. There are, however, causes for rejecting manuscripts other than lack of space.

Plethora of Material on One Subject

A plethora of material on the subject may be the reason for the return of papers on that subject—a situation likely to arise when a new treatment or theory is introduced or during and immediately following an epidemic of some disease. The introduction of arsphenamine, the sulfonamides, penicillin, streptomycin and the corticosteroids was followed by innumerable papers on those subjects. The tonsils and tonsillectomy, and especially instruments used in performing tonsillectomies, have in the past been sadly overworked subjects. At various times endocrines, cancer, vitamins and medical economics have been the subjects in vogue. More recently biochemistry, viruses, and the nervous system have been subjects of great interest.

Fancies vs. Facts

Conspicuous among the returned manuscripts are the productions of theorists who, without scientific knowledge but purely on the basis of mental gymnastics, claim that they have solved problems. Unfortunately, some physicians will discuss scientific questions although they are wholly ignorant of the fundamental and elementary principles. Such papers usually are returned with the suggestion, circumspectly phrased, that an ounce of fact is worth a ton of theory. Every physician has the right to express opinions, to advance theories and to make known his discoveries. But the reader also has his rights, and the editor must regard these rights as paramount. The reader depends on the editor not to publish fiction for fact or to publish fallacies which he, the reader, is not qualified to detect. The editor is supposed to have a knowledge of the author and his dependability that the reader cannot have.

Again and again papers have announced the discovery of a bacterial causative agent for an apparently noninfectious disease. If the author is a man of well-earned national repute and a frequent contributor to medical literature, consideration must be given to the publication. But far more harm is done in the publication of fallacious matter than in procrastinating with, or rejecting, a dozen papers offering new theories and new evidence which may be of value but which are not convincing.

Often a writer wishes to bring his manuscript personally to the editor and to stand by while the editor reads, with explanations of portions that the editor may not understand. Authors should remember that they cannot personally accompany each copy of the periodical to each subscriber.

The Medical Society Address

One of the chief causes of the over-abundance of medical periodical literature undoubtedly is the publication of papers that were written not for publication but to be read before a medical society. A large percentage of articles in medical journals are of this type. Frequently such articles are based on textbooks or on easily accessible literature and do not contain original observation, new thought or record of experience. They may review a subject in a more or less complete form and thus be useful to read before a society, since they constitute a basis for a general discussion; but they may not be worth publishing. As a rule, they are not so well thought out nor so carefully written as are papers prepared especially for printing. Thus they neither elevate the quality of periodical literature nor add to the knowledge of scientific medicine. The demand of medical societies for contributions to their programs is the only excuse that may be offered for the deficiencies of such manuscripts.

Specialists or consultants from urban areas frequently are invited by the smaller medical societies to present papers which in many cases are likely to be better prepared than those of members of the society, whose usual purpose is merely to open a discussion. The visitor is anxious to make a good impression. He thus brings profit not only to others but also to himself. Often, however, such papers may rightly be dubbed "potboilers." They, too, usually are written for reading, not for printing.

Frequently the secretary of a medical society sends a paper to an editor with the statement that it was received enthusiastically by the members of the society, who voted that it be submitted for publication with their approval. The editor finds, to his astonishment, that the paper is ungrammatical, discursive or verbose, or poorly organized, without sequence in argument or in arrangement of the subject. The author's presentation, his inflections and, above all, his personality were responsible for the success of the manuscript; the audience did not detect any fault and gave him applause and congratulations.

If an author is to be the only speaker, his anxiety will be not as to how briefly he can present his subject but as to how he will fill the time he has been assigned. Brevity, conciseness, the elimination of unnecessary details and the avoidance both of branching off into unrelated and irrelevant subjects and of the use of colloquial language will not give him concern. He will consider as appropriate and proper the relating of unimportant incidents in his experience; for instance, in a case report he will make an occasional aside and personal allusions. In this he will be right. But he will not be right if he submits his article for publication without modification. Common courtesy compels his audience to remain and listen until he concludes his address, but if his paper is prolix or rambling it will have few readers. When the paper is published the personal equation does not enter and the courtesy of the listener has vanished.

Many of the manuscripts rejected by medical periodicals have been returned because they were prepared for reading before a society and evidently submitted for publication without revision. A manuscript that is fit to read is sometimes fit to print, but a manuscript that is fit to print is always fit to read.

Length

An occasional reason for the return of a manuscript is its length. Like Einstein's theory as to space and time, however, length in this case is a matter of relativity. A paper of 500 words may be long; one of 5,000 may be short. The primary consideration is whether the material justifies the length. Usually manuscripts are unnecessarily long because of easily avoidable faults in construction, such as rambling, verbosity and diffuseness.

A STANDARD

Manuscripts, therefore, are rejected by discriminating editors for various reasons relating to the suitability of the material and to its general construction. Of these, by far the most important is the material; if the contribution is of value, other faults are susceptible to correction.

A manuscript should be suited to its audience. One which is

easily intelligible and interesting to biologic chemists may have little appeal to otolaryngologists. The details of a new technic for estimating uric acid will attract few general practitioners, who do not have the apparatus for performing the technic.

The standards set for papers presented to the Scientific Assembly of the American Medical Association is significant. This standard provides that papers must (1) contain and establish positively new facts, modes of practice or principles of real value, (2) embody the results of well-advised, original researches or (3) present so complete a review of the facts concerning any particular subject as to enable the reader to deduce legitimate, important conclusions from the article.

2
STYLE

James Huneker said, "Style cannot be taught. A good style is direct, plain and simple. The writer's keyboard is that humble camel, the dictionary." Quiller-Couch said it differently: "Style in writing is much the same thing as good manners in other human intercourse."

Dr. Walter R. Bett of London said in an address to the American Medical Writers' Association, "The essence of style, as I see it, is the avoidance of, one, wind, two, obscurity. Unfortunately, medicine has a vocabulary of its own, using many professional terms which, though often inelegant, have a definite meaning and unavoidably have come to stay."

FINE, OR FANCY, WRITING

"Whenever you feel an impulse to perpetrate a piece of exceptionally fine writing, obey it—whole-heartedly—and delete it before sending your manuscript to press. *Murder your darlings*," said Quiller-Couch again. "Fine writing" is not especially a fault of medical literature, yet it occurs with amazing frequency. Following are examples from manuscripts submitted for publication:

> The pragmatic verity of this physiological concept of disease is established by its usefulness:—with functional integrity our goal, the no-thoroughfare of unattainable structural integrity leaves us no longer at a therapeutic non-plus.

The above sounds like an erudite pronouncement, but does it mean anything?

> But what of the child? Who has championed its rights? Summoned against its will or without its consent into this world of trouble, pain, sickness and finally death, what Rousseau or Voltaire shall sound the

tocsin, and call upon the infant muling and puking in the nurse's arms, to demand that its own mother shall give it that lactic fluid that is its primal right. Bid it howl like all the heads of Cerberus against being condemned to partake of milk of cerulean hue contaminated by *Bacillus bulgaricus* prescribed by some adolescent and ardent disciple of Aesculapius. What Danton or Robespierre shall band together the sansculotte toddlers so that they may not be torn from the kindly face of mother earth, washed and dressed and sent to kindergarten where all of their play is so scientifically arranged by followers of Pestalozzi and Froebel that good fairies are unknown to them, and a "primrose beside a mossy bank, is to them but a primrose, nothing more." Where they are taught, like the clown in Lady Browning's poem, "to pick simples, turning a broad back to the glory of the stars."

The author meant this seriously, for he wished to promote nursing of babies by their mothers. It was part of a presidential address before a serious gathering and apparently was accumulated largely from Bartlett's *Familiar Quotations*.

The specificity and mathematical exactness of its effects in given dosages of which Ehrlich dreamed has gone glimmering among the pitfalls of spirochetal individuality and variation in human susceptibility.

Here the error is not so obvious; it lies in the use of words which sound extraordinarily well but which do not apply and therefore are confusing. Note "glimmering" and "pitfalls."

A florid, roseate style, full of polysyllabic, metaphorical phraseology, distracts the reader's attention. Seldom is it necessary in scientific writing to employ other than simple English terms to express an idea or to state a fact. The medical reader is acquainted with technical terms, but one should not take advantage of this to make the sentence unduly polysyllabic. The use of literary allusions to give the impression of learning, especially when the allusions are incorrect or have no direct relation to the subject discussed, is a frequent fault. For example:

The neurologist, with all of his knowledge of minutest anatomy, was for years like the "man who stood on the bridge at midnight," not dreaming the dreams of a Longfellow but soliloquizing after the manner of the cynic on the vanity of all earthly things when, lo, the voice of the syphilographer first cried from out of the darkness: "Fear not, for I am with you always."

The following statement was submitted exactly as set forth here, with the request that it be published as written or returned to its author:

> By septaecemia I mean any virulent infection where pathogenic organisms together with their toxines invade the constitution; septic blood poison, not less, no other.
>
> I speak for free and unlimited drainage, as free and unlimited as successful fortification against the savage on-rush of the enemy indicates. These drainages should be of gause soaked in pure iodine. They should be renewed frequently until victory is assured. Pure, full strength iodine brought thus to impregnate the infected area, will diffuse itself as will no other remedy except terpentine, which is its only legitimate substitute. This brings it into close hand-to-hand combat with the invading enemy; they are immediately destroyed and there toxines nutralized. Iodine is so far superior to any other remedy in this conflict, that none other need be mentioned. It is the Field Marshall; the General Grant of such battles. The best of any other remedy save terpentine, it is to iodine in such battles as a popgun is to a machine gun.

It was returned!

And here a dermatologist, confronted by a request for an address on a special occasion, took his pen in hand, tore up his books on rhetoric and grammar and spoke freely:

> When Richet, whose talents were capitalized by the winnings of a Mediterranean gambler instead of by the sanctified swag of a field marshal of industry, discovered the nature of anaphylaxis, he started medical imagination on another flight into the hectic realms of hit or miss. The phenomenon he discovered was definite. It meant something, and still does. But the lily has been gilded by countless clumsy brushes, and the ultimate daub is allergy, God save the mark, as interpreted and applied today. The metaphors in this paragraph have been mixed intentionally in order to symbolize how confused a simple thing can become when the human mind strikes its stride. For a moment let us travel backwards the path of medical history, and note the sign posts. First a philosophy based on the humors which colored etiological concepts until the middle ages. Then the great intellectual jolt by Harvey, a reveille that bounced Galenism out of its ancestral coma. Thereafter a scramble of ideas preeminently the doctrine of the diathesis, gouty in England, dartrous in France. Another jolt, Pasteur; another, Virchow; another, Ehrlich. Parasites, cell pathology, immunity! Is it remarkable that the medical world went crazy? And then Richet.
>
> And in the train of all these, first a germ for every illness, then a

cell change for every nuance of illness, then an antibody in no man's land attempting a truce between the parasite and cell, to the ultimate victory of health; then a catchpenny word, catchpenny because a great idea, that of anaphylaxis, was Kiwanised out of all recognition by the Rotarian minded in a world wide Gopher Prairie, while the instructed could only sit back in stunned contemplation. But a bit of optimism arose in them as they mused with Villon, "where are the snows of yesteryear?"

And these snows, what are they? Humoral pathology in all its classic ingenuousness, the miasma, the mesmeric moon, allopathy, homeopathy, the spleen, black bile, yellow bile, dark blood, phlegm, the diatheses, malaria, idiosyncrasy, susceptibility, hypersusceptibility, all once were dignified in speculative etiology. Where are they today? And tomorrow, where will be focal infections, where, allergy? "Non omnis moriar," sang Horace, nor will these either entirely die, but when they have survived the purgatory of misconstruction, their lambent spirits, resurrected, will lead medicine onward after the fools and opportunists have had their fling.

If ever a subject warranted such hyperbole, allergy would; but one's mind and ears have become hypersensitive to hyperbole.

Among typical violations of the rules against fine writing are the following usages:

"Gentleman" instead of "man."
"Inaugurate" instead of "begin."
"The patient sustained an injury" instead of "The patient was injured."
"Canine" instead of "dog."

VERBOSITY

Verbosity is a blemish in the writing of most people—one that makes reading tedious, mars diction and wastes space. This fault can be overcome easily, but in most instances not efficiently until after the paper has been written. Unless you have tried it, you will be astonished at the number of words, phrases, clauses, sentences and, occasionally, paragraphs that can be deleted without affecting the meaning. Deletions of unnecessary words always improve grammatical construction and style of expression and facilitate reading with understanding.

Quiller-Couch, in his book entitled *On the Art of Writing*,[1] devoted a chapter to verbiage. Here is one of his illustrations:

---
[1] Quiller-Couch, Arthur: *On the Art of Writing.* New York, G. P. Putnam's Sons, 1916.

> A clerk of a Board of Guardians had to record a minute relative to the burial of a pauper. The minute reads:
> "In the case of John Jenkins, deceased, the coffin provided was of the usual character."

Sir Arthur pulled the sentence to pieces. It is superfluous to say that Jenkins is deceased; the fact that he needs a coffin is sufficient evidence. "In the case of" is superfluous, for Jenkins did not have a case; he had, and needed, only a coffin. The coffin was not "of the usual character," for coffins have no character. The clerk should have said, "John Jenkins was provided with the usual coffin."

An article by A. G. Macdonell, published in the London *Lancet,* complimented Winston Churchill, who in an interval between organizing the defense of the British Empire and winning the war, found time to send a little memorandum to his colleagues in the Government, asking them to alter their style of writing the English language. In his letter Mr. Churchill insisted that all official documents and memorandums should be short. He wrote, "Let us have an end to such phrases as 'It is also of importance to bear in mind the following considerations,' and again, 'consideration should be given to the possibility of carrying into effect . . .'"

Mr. Macdonell continued, quoting: "'the answer is in the affirmative' will now have to give place to the old-fashioned Anglo-Saxon word 'yes.' The phrase, 'considering all the circumstances, it would probably be correct to answer this question in a contrary fashion,' will have to give place to the old simple 'no.'

"What a lot of beautiful phrases are going to be scrapped because of the Prime Minister," said Mr. Macdonell. "'With regard to the question as to whether,' for example. That will have to go. 'In view of all the circumstances arising in and from.' That is another. Then there is, 'While admitting that the opinions expressed in our letter of the 24th ult. undoubtedly were expressed in that letter, we cannot admit that those opinions were in any way binding on anyone connected with this department.'"

Here are specimens from real life—from manuscripts submitted for publication:

> I do not hesitate to say that in my opinion the gland in this case should not have been removed.

Style

The first seven words are space takers. I have characterized this as a "running start." The author fills in with words while assembling a thought. The shorter sentence, "In this case, in my opinion, the gland should not have been removed," was printed. Possibly "in my opinion" also might have been deleted.

This from another author:

> It has been a mooted question in the minds of microbiologists whether the gonococcus possesses a capsule.

The difference between a mooted question and one that is not mooted is problematic. "In the minds of microbiologists" carries the idea that only microbiologists are concerned. The sentence was improved by divesting it of verbiage, and when printed it read:

> It has been a question whether the gonococcus possesses a capsule.

The purist would have modified this still more and mentioned the microbiologist, making it read:

> Microbiologists question whether the gonococcus possesses a capsule.

This from an article describing an apparatus:

> Physicians who have been using radium needles will readily appreciate the difficulties encountered in threading them.

"Who have been," "will readily" and "encountered" were deleted, and the sentence revised to read:

> Physicians who use radium needles realize the difficulty of threading them.

The introduction to a case report read:

> The following case is reported on account of the unusual occurrence of *Ascaris lumbricoides* in an adult of sufficient quantity to cause obstruction of small intestine, necessitating resection of intestine.
>
> Miss R. of A———, Ala., referred to me by Dr. M. S. of ———, aged 36, single, admitted to the hospital at Albany, Ala., Nov. 6, 1947, suffering with intense pain in the abdomen, in the right hypochondriac region. She was a poorly nourished woman and suffering great shock and presented all the symptoms of an intestinal obstruction.

The first paragraph could be omitted by entitling the paper: "*Ascaris lumbricoides* Causing Obstruction of Intestine in an Adult: Report of a Case in Which Resection Was Necessary."

The report contains a large number of unnecessary words, from the point of view both of good writing and of facts necessary to adequate presentation. With the unnecessary words bracketed for omission, the report appears:

> Miss R., [of A———, Ala., referred to me by Dr. M. S. of ———] aged 36, [single, admitted to the hospital at Albany, Ala.] was seen on Nov. 6, 1947, suffering with [intense] abdominal pain in the right hypochondriac region, [She was a poorly nourished woman and suffering great shock and presented all the symptoms of] apparently due to intestinal obstruction.

POOR GRAMMAR

The modern physician presumably has had the advantage of education in a university. Therefore, when an editor receives from a physician a manuscript in which sentence after sentence reveals grammatical faults that would disgrace a seventh-grade student, he must surmise that the author has failed to give proper attention to the writing of his article.

Here are some examples from manuscripts:

> In meningococcic meningitis the optic nerve is involved as a perineuritis, there is not a papilloedema in contradistinction to the papilloedema the result of pressure from distention of the optic prolongation of the third ventricle pressing on the chiasmal cystern as occurs in meningitis of pyogenic origin.
>
> In general the larger abscesses had the higher counts, with one exception, 23 days after an unoperated appendicitis with 14,400 white blood cells and 3,000 cc. of pus.
>
> There were four cases of appendicitis, none of which had been operated except for a pelvic abscess in one.
>
> Medulloblastomas develop almost invariably in children taking their origin just over the fourth ventricle.
>
> Scabies is also a frequency with the Negro, for he fails to realize the severity and the laxity of consulting a physician, resulting in rapid and wide dissemination of this highly contagious parasitic skin infection to others, and in many instances the starting of an epidemic.
>
> Her pelvis had been injured by being thrown from a motorcycle.
>
> Williams states that he induced the animals to take the hydrocarbon by licking it off a glass rod.

Here is a specimen of highly confused grammar from a chairman's address before one of the scientific sections of the American Medical Association:

We have had a sister specialized field, that of Ophthalmology. Very few of the older men still practicing but whom earlier in their careers did not embrace both fields, and I am not sure but when after they gravitated to one or the other they were not better men for having at one time applied their knowledge to both. There is something to be said against narrowing one's horizon too much. This may be debatable but there is an economic side that is not to be disputed. There are communities which are entitled to good service but are not large enough to support physicians devoting their attention to only ophthalmology or otolaryngology. Statistical studies are lacking but the American Board of Otolaryngology some four years ago put out a questionnaire upon which the secretary, Dr. W. P. Wherry, informs me warranted them to conclude, etc.

A dermatologist perpetrated this atrocity:

In conclusion, realizing the conflicting data that can be gathered from the literature on the subject of the treatment of lues co-existing with pulmonary tuberculosis, a program for such therapy has been presented, which, so far indicates that syphilis in the presence of pulmonary tuberculosis can be treated and, though modified, treated adequately according to accepted standards of adequate treatment without any deleterious effect on the pulmonary lesion if caution and rigid scrutiny are enforced at all times, using all laboratory aids available including radiography and providing nothing, no matter how trivial, is dismissed without diligent investigation.

Here are further examples from manuscripts:

Gonorrhea is extremely common due to the same attitude of mind in that same is not a disease requiring no treatment, but speaks of it as female trouble, and continues to journey along with his discharge until it has subsided, to return at a future time after it has become chronic.

The use of a syringe introduced with the plunger down and suction made at different depths should be done.

The history of these cases are usually rather obscure and are slow in their progress, which usually effectually wipes out the connection between them.

After a search in literature I can't find a case of General Paralysis in a woman that gave birth to an apparently normal child, which after five months shows no stigmata of syphilis, and where the mother before delivery was demented and partially oriented has improved so much in five months after delivery that she is oriented in all spheres, carries on a fairly well connected conversation and takes care of her house satisfactorily.

Such results should make physicians enthusiastic not only to do their part to make children safe from diphtheria, but also to make the children of the communities safe in which they live.

These horrible examples of what a medical author may perpetrate are offered merely as exhibits, with the hope that the reader will be impressed with a necessity of carefully reading each sentence of his own manuscript to determine its grammatical purity. Long, involved, ungrammatical sentences make the sequence of ideas difficult or impossible to follow, and papers containing them are seldom read to the end.

Most common grammatical errors found in articles submitted for publication are the following:

Affect and Effect

These two words frequently are interchanged. "Affect" means *to act on;* "effect," *to bring about.*

The following quotations are from an editorial by William H. Woglom in *Cancer Research, 2*:846, Dec., 1942:

QUESTION AS TO. Fowler calls this an ugly and needless formula.
The question arises as to whether the tumors were caused by the injections. [Wrong.]
The question arises whether or not the tumors were caused by the injections. [Right.]

AS LARGE, OR LARGER, THAN. This is a common fallacy. A moment's reflection will show that when the little afterthought and its enclosing commas have been deleted, "as large, or larger, than a plum" becomes "as large than a plum," which is manifestly absurd. The correct expression is "as large as, or larger than, a plum." This paragraph does not condone the careless habit of comparing the size of a lesion with that of some familiar object. Actual dimensions, expressed in the metric system, are, of course, preferred.

DIFFERENT THAN. The expression "different than" enjoys an enormous popularity; nevertheless, it is wrong. "Different from" is right.

Restrictive and Nonrestrictive Elements

Woolley offers a useful rule for determining whether a given clause is nonrestrictive (may be set off by commas) or restrictive (must not be set off by commas). He says that if the main assertion of the sentence retains its meaning when the clause is omitted, the clause is nonrestrictive. But if the omission changes the sense of the main assertion, the clause is restrictive. For example: "The directions that appeared on the label were wrong" (restrictive). "The directions, which had been meant for another patient, were wrong" (nonrestrictive). "Prefer those words which are short" (restrictive). "He quoted those words, which he had always remembered" (nonrestrictive).

CORRELATIVES

Conjunctions that are used in pairs are called correlatives. Examples are: not only . . . but also . . . ; both . . . and . . .; either . . . or . . . ; neither . . . nor . . . ; not . . . or . . . ; whether . . . or . . .

These conjunctions should be followed by parallel elements; if a predicate follows one, a predicate should follow the other. If a prepositional phrase follows one, a prepositional phrase should follow the other.

The sentence "He was not only courteous to rich customers but also to poor ones" is faulty, as pointed out by Greever and Jones in their *Handbook of Writing*. The phrases intended to be balanced against each other are "to rich customers" and "to poor ones." Instead, the word "courteous" is balanced against "to poor ones." The correct form is "He was courteous not only to rich customers but also to poor ones."

The following is incorrect: "She could neither make up her mind to go nor could she decide to stay." The correct form is: "She could neither make up her mind to go nor decide to stay." Or, "She could not make up her mind either to go or to stay."

One should not write "I talked both with Brown and Miller." One conjunction is followed by a preposition and the other by a noun. Correct usage is "I talked with both Brown and Miller." Or, "I talked both with Brown and with Miller."

SLANG

Medicine is a dignified science. The attitude of the medical profession and of the public toward a scientific paper is dependent largely on the spirit in which the paper is written. Much of the dignity accruing to medicine today is dependent on the fact that physicians usually have presented their contributions in language suited to the subject. Few editors care to publish discussions of serious matters offered in a tone of levity. The following are examples from papers submitted for publication, indicating that the language of the street or of the preparation room is not suited to the discussion of surgical technic or of medical practice:

> We have long passed the stage where any operation is considered a success if the patient survives, and in this particular one, where lots of blood and two or three chunks of tissue extracted from the patient's pharynx means good throat surgery.
> A surgeon may be a "whiz" in the abdomen or in grafting bones, but a proverbial "bull in a china shop" in the throat.
> The G. U. man has appropriated the term "syphilis," but the fact that the initial lesion is frequently on the genitals does not make the disease other than systemic.
> He will not attempt an iridectomy or cataract extraction, but seemingly feels "T. & A.'s" are "duck soup" where as a matter of fact the finished specialist realizes there is little difference in the skill required for all when well done.
> I recall one of my first stricture cases (a woman) who had gone the rounds for three years. She spent a week in a hospital in Richmond, seeking a diagnosis. She did not have symptoms referable to the urinary tract and her physician did not cystoscope her. She then went to Asheville for a six weeks dietary treatment, and so on. She finally came to one of my associates, who requested cystoscopy. We were unable to get a filiform into the right ureter. We cystoscoped her every day for five days, finally getting a No. 2 olive-tipped bougie to enter.
> This was a strangulated affair of four days' duration.

KEEPING SAME POINT OF VIEW THROUGHOUT THE PAPER

Tenses

Writers often skip from one tense to another, even within a paragraph, which may confuse the reader. Tenses should be consistent, except that scientific truths are expressed in the present tense. For example, one would say, "A diagnosis of appendicitis was considered, as the appendix is sometimes eccentrically located." To say *"was* sometimes" here would be absurd.

Woglom emphasizes that good reason does not exist for describing experiments in the past tense and microscopic morphology in the present, though this is common practice. Perhaps the safest method is to keep to the past tense in all descriptive matter. In the publications of the American Medical Association the past tense is used for verbs of saying or recording, except in reviews of the literature covering a single year, where the author may use the present tense if he prefers it.

A related difficulty lies in the expressions "he believed" and "he believes." It may be impossible to determine whether the view cited is still held and therefore whether "he believes" is correct. "He believed," on the other hand, may imply that the opinion has been abandoned. The difficulty can be avoided, as a rule, by changing the verb of thinking to a verb of saying, so that, for instance, "Brown considered" becomes "Brown expressed the opinion." In reviews of recent literature with verbs of saying in the present tense and in papers in which an author discusses recent work by men whose opinions he obviously knows well, "he believes" is, of course, permissible.

Singular and Plural Forms

Serious misunderstanding as well as an impression that an author is careless may be caused by failure to retain the same approach throughout a paper, especially in regard to the use of singular and plural forms. You begin by speaking of "the eye" and "the kidney" and later find yourself mentioning "the frontal lobes" and "the lungs." Often a manuscript editor working on a paper which has been accepted finds himself confronted by phrases such as these: "The fundus seemed normal . . . . In the scleras and corneas . . . ." When organs are spoken of in a general sense, they should be referred to consistently in either the singular or the plural, and when specific observations are described, it should be stated whether one (if so, which) or both of the organs were examined or were affected.

Even more confusion is caused by a paragraph such as the following, which was taken from a manuscript received for publication:

> In the thorax the intercostal or phrenic nerves may give rise to a neurofibroma, these often attaining a considerable size. The benignity of the tumor makes surgical removal a most satisfying procedure, and one who is familiar with operations on the thoracic wall and in the chest cavities has little difficulty in completely enucleating these growths. . . . An example of neurofibroma of an intercostal nerve is seen in case 21. . . . The relative softness of the lungs of other intrathoracic structures often allows one of these neoplasms to readily expand and assume a great size. Harrington has reported 14 cases of mediastinal or intrathoracic perineural fibroblastomata, and his success in treating these lesions again emphasizes the desirability of recognizing such benign growths and attempting surgical extirpation. Of 46 various intrathoracic tumors removed at operation, this author classified 14 of them as of nerve sheath origin, and 10 of these occurred in the posterior mediastinum. The presence of a neurofibroma in the posterior mediastinum and in the neck may lead to dumb-bell-shaped tumors which pass through into the spinal canal.

A similar faulty construction, not quite so confusing but equally illogical and more frequent, follows:

> In these cases the lesions [it is understood that there was one in each case] began on the face and extended downward, finally covering the neck and the chest.

The author may argue that if there are cases, there are also lesions, rather than a lesion. But are there not also faces, necks and chests? Moreover, if another author should quote only this passage, the reader of the quotation might be forced to consult the original article to determine whether more than one lesion was present in each case.

There can be no confusion if the sentence reads:

> In these cases the lesion began on the face and extended downward, finally covering the neck and the chest.

USE OF NOUNS AS ADJECTIVES

Practically all important publications avoid excessive use of nouns as adjectives to modify other nouns. This policy should not be interpreted as a series of "Thou shalt not's" with regard to specific phrases. The tendency to eliminate adjectives from the language by supplanting them with nouns should be avoided.

The following excerpts from an article by Lord Dunsany in the *Atlantic Monthly*[2] state the problem admirably:

> The decay that is affecting our language is taking place among adjectives; so much so that many of these necessary things have already died. One cannot prove that an adjective is dead merely because in so many hundred pages it never appears; the proof is when the need of that particular adjective arises and it is not used, a noun being thrown in to take its place, as a sheet of paper may stop a hole in a window in the absence of a pane of glass.
>
> If you read of "a strange man in an expensive car," that is no proof that other adjectives equally suitable are dead; but if you read of "a mystery man in a luxury car" that proves that the adjectives "mysterious" and "luxurious" have decayed away, for no one would otherwise use this lumber of nouns. There is, of course, no lack of meaning in "a mystery man in a luxury car"; only a lack of grace. I imagine that hundreds of things had names among savages a thousand years before those graces appeared by which the Romans, for instance, built their sentences; and I think that the deepness of the German forests, which the legions did not easily penetrate, is probably responsible for the German tendency to use heaps of nouns to this day, a clumsiness unknown in France and Italy.
>
> When meaning disappears from modern sentences is the moment that a third noun is added to the heap, or even an honest adjective; as for instance, if we were to write "a great luxury man," it would not be quite clear whether we were intending a man who lived in great luxury or whether a luxury man of large size. If instead of the adjective "great" we have yet another noun, the confusion is liable to be even worse. There are no landmarks to guide one through this confusion, for in a single copy of the *Times* I read two advertisements: the first of them spoke of "best position seats"—obviously the hyphen, which was not there, should be imagined between the first word and the second; but there are no rules for this clumsy game, because the other advertisement spoke of a "great equality myth," and in that case the hyphen had to be understood between the second word and the third.
>
> It may be quite clear to my readers why the hyphen should have come in each case where I have said that it should; but I have had the advantage of reading the context, and have worked it out in that way. The alternative to reading the context is to know exactly which of several ambiguities the writer intends with his row of nouns, and for

---

[2]Dunsany, Edward: Decay in the language. *Atlantic Monthly, 157:*360-362, March, 1936.

this purpose you must obviously know just what he intends to say. Does not this mean that in the language of jumbled nouns you can only say what everyone knows already? Then the writer with something new to say will not be understood, even when he has got a hearing.

GOBBLEDYGOOK IN MEDICAL WRITING

"Gobbledygook" is an American colloquialism defined as "speech or exposition that is obscured by excessive use of technical terminology, involved sentences, and big words."

In a letter to the editor of the *American Journal of Psychiatry* (Gobbledygook in psychiatric writing. *American Journal of Psychiatry*, December, 1951, p. 474), a writer signing himself L. K. said:

> New words and concise delineations cannot be avoided and are often indispensable. But involved, long-winded, redundant, tautological, "obfuscating" language, to which the name gobbledygook has been applied, can, and should, be avoided. In analyzing some of the glaring transgressions, it is not always easy to distinguish between literary depositions of muddled thinkers and clumsy phrasing by clear thinkers.
>
> A few years ago, *The New Yorker* picked up a passage from an article in a psychiatric journal. The attitudes and manners shown by the British in tea drinking, eating, smoking, and general behavior suggested to the author that "it is possible to detect in the English, taken as a nation, the cultivation of oral sucking impulses and the inhibition of aggression of a more direct and brutal type, from biting onwards. Given certain circumstances, these repressions are lifted, and the super-ego is able to tolerate the exercise of the corresponding functions." The amused editor asked: "One lump or two lumps, Doctor?"
>
> Here is a passage—a sentence longer even than the yawn it may evoke—taken from a book that has had a wide circulation:
>
> "If the restitution required of the individual necessitates a very strong sense of constructive omnipotence—as, for instance, that he shall make complete restitution towards both parents and towards his brothers and sisters, etc., and, by displacement, towards other objects and even the entire world—then, whether he will do great things in life and whether the development of his ego and of his sexual life will be successful, or whether he will fall a victim to severe inhibitions, will partly depend upon the strength of his ego and the degree of his adaptation to reality which regulates those imaginary requirements, and partly upon whether the tasks laid upon him are too exacting and the discrepancy between his destructive and constructive omnipotence exceeds a certain limit."

It should be emphasized that the majority of psychiatrists write clearly and sensibly. But there is still too much gobbledgook and too much "excess ideological baggage," as Whitehorn called it in his presidential address. The reasons for this are undoubtedly numerous and complex. A few points, however, suggest themselves immediately:

1. Some of us seem to fear simplicity lest it be mistaken for mediocrity.

2. There seems to be some apprehension that the public will not be impressed by clear and direct statements made in everyday language. After all, everybody can say things simply, and isn't the specialist under obligation to display his erudition for the sake of professional prestige?

3. The advent of the "deep" psychologies has instilled in some of us a dread of being branded as "superficial" if we do not couch our talk in some sort of professional jargon. This has led some to the pseudo-logical conclusion that a goodly portion of balderdash will assure one's reputation as an expert in "depth."

4. One-sided training in specialized techniques has caused some of us to overrate their value out of all proportion to the broad field of psychiatry. Limited experience has resulted in a limited form of expression, often compensated by garrulous repetitiousness. Douglas M. Kelley, in a recent publication in this Journal, has brilliantly demonstarted the abuses of Rorschach interpretations through "generalities, multiordinal terms, superficial description, and temperament depictions that can apply to anybody." Similar criticism can be leveled at the practitioners of other restricted methods applied out of context with clinical and social "reality."

I have collected a few examples of gobbledygook from recently published books and articles. Some of these follow:

... during its earliest years the child thinks primarily in terms of visual images. The parents and their substitutes come to form composite images in the mind of the child, and these images or "imagos" persist for a lifetime. [Who needs that word "imagos"?]

The impulse neurosis adds nothing new to our study of psychodynamics. It combines the ego-syntonic character of psychopathy with the ritualistic, circumscribed symptomatology of compulsive obsessive state. [Isn't that clear?]

There is little heuristic value in erecting a specific hierarchy of the neuroses and psychoses as correlated to a multiple stage account of the development and vicissitudes of the libido. Instead it can be contended on both theoretic and clinical grounds (a) that the so-called libidinal stages of development have a temporal existence only in so far as the growing infant becomes physiologically capable of expressing them, and (b) that in later life the "psychological" counterparts of these libidinal organ-cathexes overlap and mingle in a way that makes analysis of complex psychotic reactions in terms of simple "orality," "anality" or "genitality" analogous to committing mayhem on the facts. [As they say in the international congresses, "please translate."]

One glossary of psychiatric terms yields such weird words as:
homilophobia—a fear of sermons
necromimesis—acting as though dead
osphresiophilia—a morbid fascination with odors
peniaphobia—a morbid dread of poverty

For some time I have argued with publishers that a book which requires a glossary should be declined on the ground that it needs to be thoroughly edited, if not rewritten.

Big words, complex sentences and extraordinary diction seem to have become the ordinary language of psychiatry.

ACQUIRING A GOOD STYLE

The formula for acquiring a good literary style has two ingredients: reading and practice. Extensive reading of the works of good writers invariably will increase the vocabulary and improve the style.

A style that flows attractively from the pen comes only as the result of much practice. "A well constructed phrase," said Flaubert, "adapts itself to the rhythm of respiration." Clauses and phrases of even length permit proper emphasis.

Write and rewrite; rewrite again and then revise!

Dr. Allen Gregg, Director for the Medical Sciences, Rockefeller Foundation, said in a commencement address delivered at the Jefferson Medical College in 1943:

> The common level of medical and scientific writing in our professional books and journals already constitutes the most serious internal limitation to medical education and research. The usual level of professional writing is painful not merely to editors. Even after passing editorial filters, the virus of wretched writing can inflame, insult, and exhaust a clear-minded man. Such writing is verbose and repetitious. It is awkward and tiresome. What time it can spare from being vague it devotes to being inaccurate. By sheer carelessness of phraseology, the author belies his probable meaning by actual misstatement. Such writing defeats the very purpose of communication—to convey information clearly. The amount of carelessly written papers overwhelms every one; the quality debases the standards of beginners

and the quantity obstructs and exhausts every honest and discriminating worker. I know of no editor of any medical journal who cannot at any time testify to the sheer incompetence of the writing in an inexcusable proportion of the papers submitted for publication. And even with the benefit of hours of editorial improvement, the medical literature of today exemplifies all too fully the biological adage that life is choked by its own secretions.

3
THE SUBJECT AND THE MATERIAL

A DISTINCT CHANGE is apparent in the type of papers appearing in medical journals in 1970 compared with those of 1905. The therapeutic articles of the past, replete with favorite prescriptions, have given way to scientific contributions on therapeutic methods, pharmacology, pathology, etiology, methods of diagnosis and prophylaxis. The difference can be appreciated only by those who were in practice in the earlier period or by those who will compare the journals of that time with the present.

Dr. Charles Singer,[1] in his essay on "Greek Biology and Its Relation to the Rise of Modern Biology," described a complete contribution of the best type in modern scientific literature.

> The author begins by pointing out a gap in knowledge. . . . Having stated his problem, he reviews the efforts made by others to illumine this dark place in knowledge. He points out some of their errors or decides to accept their work and base his own upon it. Perhaps he distrusts their experiments or would like to reinterpret their results. Having summarized their labours he details his own experiments and observations.
>
> But he is not able to tell us all of these. . . . Space will not permit him to tell us how he embarked on many different lines of work and abandoned them as unprofitable or too difficult, nor anything of the months or years spent in merely repeating the experience of others. He says no word of how he acquired and improved his experimental skill and technical experience. He tells merely of those developments of his work that have yielded him results. . . . When by gradual steps he had

---
[1]Singer, Charles: Greek biology and its relation to the rise of modern biology. In *Studies in the History and Method of Science.* Oxford, England, Clarendon Press, 1921, vol. 2, p. 1.

at last reached, or perhaps with the instinct of genius had more quickly discerned, a profitable direction for his investigations, he reached after a time those conclusions which his final line of work has verified and rendered more exact. It is this final process of verification that he mainly describes in his article, and it is the details of this that occupy the bulk, perhaps nineteen-twentieths or more, of all that he has to say. Then, having described these verificatory experiments, he summarizes his conclusions in a short paragraph of a few lines."

TYPES OF ARTICLES

Medical articles may be classified in definite types, including:
1. The case report.
2. The description of a new instrument.
3. The clinical note or suggestion.
4. The review of literature.
5. The essay.
6. The report of research.
7. The complete consideration of a single disease.
8. The monograph.
9. A combination of two or more of these types.

The Case Report

The foundation of clinical medical literature is the case report. A case report usually should not include a review of previous papers. If it records an instance of a rare disease or abnormality, however, a few well-chosen references may be in order.

History of the Case Report

The first case reports in medical history appeared in Edwin Smith's Surgical Papyrus (*circa* 1700 B.C.). Twelve hundred years later the Hippocratic text provided another group of medical records, including cases in surgery, medicine and obstetrics. Subsequent notable contributors have included Morgagni, Sydenham and Richard Cabot.

Technic of the Case Report

Sir John Charles, Chief Medical Officer to the Minister of Health in Great Britain, in an opening address at the First International Congress on Medical Records, London, Sept. 8, 1952, said, "Above all comes the scheduling of the facts, and the little verse of Kipling mentions most of them:

> I keep six honest serving-men (they taught me all I know),
> Their names are What and Why and When, and How and Where and Who.

A case report should tell its story in clear, straightforward, narrative style. It should not be transcribed word-for-word from original records that were hastily jotted down at the time the various events occurred. The jerky, telegraphic style of the record sheet may actually be redundant. For example:

> Patient, A178493, Giuseppe Roverano. Age 35 years. Color, white. Nationality, Italian. Occupation, laborer. Condition, married. Complaint, inflammatory rheumatism. Entered Brown Hospital, Jan. 17, 1948.

A shorter and more satisfactory description would be as follows:

> G. R., an Italian laborer aged 35, married, entered the Brown Hospital on Jan. 17, 1948, with symptoms of inflammatory rheumatism.

Laboratory and other reports made by someone other than the author, which have not been published elsewhere, should not be copied in their original form but should be edited to conform to the style of the rest of the case report.

Negative Observations and Unnecessary Material

The hospital record number is not required in a case report. While it may serve a purpose within the hospital to identify the case for the members of the staff, it means nothing to the reader. Further, it may give rise to a false impression as to the number of cases which have been observed in the institution by the physician.

Mention of observations that are unimportant or that do not bear on the clinical history of the case should be avoided. Negative results are of value in few instances, and they should be cited only when necessary. An author who reports a case of compound fracture of the femur need not bother to say that the lips, throat and ears were normal. If, however, you are reporting a case of arthritis, it may be worthwhile to say that examination of the heart did not yield observations of importance, because pathologic changes in the heart may be associated with arthritis. "Mrs. J. J., married," is redundant, for "Mrs." indicates marriage; but "Mrs. J. J., a widow," conveys additional social information that may have some bearing on the case.

In an excellent essay, "On Case Reports," Raymond Whitehead of the University of Manchester writes, "The important point is not whether a result is positive, negative or inconclusive, but whether the information bears on the case."

Elimination of all negative or irrelevant material from a report is a valuable exercise from the point of view not only of good English composition but also of scientific knowledge. The physician who is well informed will not give all the minutiae of a normal blood count or of a normal differential leukocyte count. He will not provide a perhaps highly entertaining but valueless account of the various illnesses suffered by all the members of the patient's family. He will not say that the patient had the usual illnesses of childhood, but if any of these illnesses had a bearing on the condition, he will state what the illness was and about when it occurred. The elimination of nonessential material from the case report will make a clinical picture that will be as striking as a marble bas-relief in its proper emphasis on various features and in its subduing of background.

Here are some examples of irrelevant material included in case reports. The irrelevancies are italicized.

At 11:45 p.m. near the outskirts of a small village, twenty miles away, an infant was born to a primiparous *mother on Thursday, Oct. 14, 1947. The delivery occurred on a trundle bed in a darkened corner of a room, illuminated only with a single kerosene lamp. The attending* physician, *a rural practitioner, had been with many mothers under similar circumstances. As he kneeled over to clamp, cut and ligate the cord, his hand* felt a mass lying on the front and side of the child's abdomen. The mass was soft and pliable, and *as he ran his experienced fingers over its surface* he located the cord emerging *directly* from the mass *itself.*

He carried the child over to the lamp and to his amazement there was present on its abdomen a large part of its intestine. *It was readily seen and felt through the thin transparent membrane which close* inspection revealed *to be* the cord itself enormously dilated. The intestines protruded along the course of the cord *a distance of some* 5 or 6 inches. The mass *itself* was the size of a large cocoanut.

This newly born baby was delivered in precipitate labor while the mother sat on the stool, *supported one on either side by two neighboring women.*

On my arrival at the time (a private home) all indications pointed to very unusual circumstances—I hastily entered the home and found just such a condition as stated in my opening. Collecting my wits included many things and wondering what step to make first, while going throu a sterilizing process, with the help of the husband who had arrived a short time previously I planned an examination to determine if the babe was delivered and if still alive. The husband raised the mother sufficiently to afford a hasty examination which revealed baby was delivered and was dead from drowning. We placed them in a warm bed, *the husband carrying the mother while I supported the babe. This done* I hastily divided the Funis. *Placed the babe in a warm room upon a table.*

Nowhere are negative observations more frequently encountered than in the recapitulation of autopsy records. Sometimes such reports are practically the transcript of the stenographer's record, dictated as the examination progressed. In most instances it is sufficient to present only the anatomic diagnosis, with all the pathologic conditions, and then to give in detail the description of the particular pathologic changes with which the discussion is concerned.

Confusion of Time

A common fault in case reports is indefiniteness in sequence of events as to time; it is illustrated in the following skeleton of a case report submitted for publication:

CASE 3, A. D., Feb. 8, 1947. Hairpin in the bladder and renal infection. Girl, 22 years old, first seen three years ago. Two years ago her kidney was explored. . . . A year ago this patient went to the city hospital. . . . Soon after this I heard of her as a patient with marked polyuria. . . . From the early part of the summer until August she had retention of urine and had to be catheterized. . . . Five weeks ago she allowed a friend. . . . to attempt catheterization. . . . I saw her three weeks ago and found the hairpin. . . . I was not then allowed to remove it. . . . On February 3 she told me that the day before she had had pain in the left renal region. . . . Examination next day showed marked cystitis. The pin was removed. . . . Within four days. . . . the patient was discharged.

January 1948. Two weeks after leaving the hospital another pin was found in the bladder.

And here is another example:

He was born and lived in Turkey until he was 12, when he came to the United States. He spent two years in Boston, and the remainder of the time in California. He had had malaria ten years ago and typhoid two years ago. About four years ago his skin began to itch whenever he became warm.

As a paper may not be published for months after it is prepared, the time should be stated specifically instead of being referred to as three, five or nine months or years ago.

Tense

Tenses should be used consistently. A frequent error occurs when the author follows a case report with a description of a pathologic specimen or of a section viewed under the microscope. Often the history of the case is given in the past tense and the pathologic report in the present tense. These should be uniform. The simplest way usually is to use the past tense throughout.

In the description of observations that have been continued, it is logical to regard the time of writing as the present and to say, for instance, "At the of writing, the patient is well."

In the summary of a paper, the present tense should be used, as in the following sentence: "A case of myxedema is reported, and the literature is reviewed."

Coined Abbreviations

In many institutions certain abbreviations are customarily used in case records; this is excusable, for it saves space and makes reference easy for those who know what the abbreviations mean. In material for publication, abbreviations should be avoided, and the general use of original or coined abbreviations should not be tolerated. "W.D. & N." for "well developed and nourished." "H. & L.O.K." signifying "heart and lungs normal" and "L.L.L.N.R." for "left lower lobe no rales" are abominations. The manuscript editor who is confronted with such hieroglyphics can sympathize with the diagnosis "G.O.K." which, it is said, appeared on many case records in hospitals during the war, signifying "God only knows." Abbreviations not in dictionaries or in ordinary textbooks are permissible only in tables; there, if not obvious, they should be explained in footnotes. Such abbreviations as ACTH for adrenocorticotropic hormone come into the language but may be replaced by a name like corticotropin or the trade name Acthar.®

Form of the Report

The simple case report may begin at once with the history and record or, preferably, may be introduced with a statement of why the author considers it desirable to report the case. If the latter method is followed, the author will aid the reader and the manuscript editor by clearly indicating the separation in the following manner:

> There is no record of chronic poisoning from potassium nitrate in standard works on toxicology or therapeutics, nor does a fairly extensive search of the literature reveal any report of such poisoning.

REPORT OF CASE

> A farmer aged 57, whose general health had always been excellent, was first seen by me on Feb. 20, 1947. He appeared acutely ill....

In the report of a case of any length, the description may be broken up by side headings. Paragraphs may be devoted to the patient's history, family history, physical examination, laboratory examination, course, results and, if any, postmortem observations.

In longer manuscripts, in which several or many cases are briefly reported merely as a matter of record, a single paragraph may be given to each case.

The Description of a New Instrument

Ordinarily an instrument should be described in as few words as possible, depending largely on the accompanying illustrations of the device or apparatus to tell the story. A photograph of the device usually is better than a freehand drawing, although a drawing by a competent artist is more easily reproduced. A diagrammatic line drawing and a photograph of the device in use generally are most satisfactory. The publication of a description of an apparatus that has not been manufactured and used is unwarranted.

The Clinical Note or Suggestion

In the course of his practice, a physician frequently discovers minor clinical signs and symptoms of importance, shortcuts in procedure, bizarre occurrences or similar matters of general interest that are worth publishing. They may not merit a thorough report; rather, they may be covered in letters to the editors or in brief clinical suggestions occupying a paragraph. Such suggestions or practical paragraphs are read by almost every reader, whereas many would pay little or no attention to a long article.

The Review of Literature

One of the most valuable—and sometimes the most useless, depending on how it is prepared—types of contribution is the review of knowledge on a given subject. If the review is made by one who is familiar with the literature and who has had sufficient experience to select with judgment and to discard with even more care, the contribution may be important. If, however, the work is done by an assistant who has been instructed to obtain references to the available literature on the subject and to arrange these in chronologic or some other order, it is likely to be hodgepodge and of wearisome length. In the course of a brief article on such a subject as tuberculosis, syphilis or influenza during an epidemic abstracts of all that has been written cannot be included.

The Essay

Manuscripts of the essay type include presidential addresses, forecasts as to the future of medicine and discussions of the economic problems and the social status of the physician—more or less exhaustive discussions of selected subjects in which physicians are interested as citizens and as professional men rather than as scientists. They are obviously more literary than the usual contributions, and the physician may allow himself a latitude in literary allusion, diction and personal reference not permissible in the ordinary scientific paper. The published addresses of Sir William Osler, Sir Clifford Allbutt, S. Weir Mitchell, Oliver Wendell Holmes, William S. Thayer, Harvey Cushing, Da Costa and William B. Bean are examples of this type.

The Report of Research

No better outline of the form to be followed in a report of medical research is available than that by Singer, described in the quotation at the beginning of this chapter. Emphasis may be placed again on the necessity of rigid elimination of nonessentials. The problem should be stated clearly; the literary references should bear directly on the problem; the protocols of experiments should include only experiments that yielded actual information; clinical records and autopsy reports should be pruned religiously; there should be a well-organized summary, and the conclusions should be succinct and include only statements that are warranted by previous knowledge and the present observations.

One of the most common faults is duplication. Frequently a report of research is accompanied by extensive charts and tabulations that repeat material brought out in the text. Often a paper is received in which the observations are fully stated in the protocols of the experiments, summed up in a running account in the summary, restated and resummed up in extensive tables and again pictured graphically in intricate charts. The procedure is much like presenting a diner with three desserts composed of strawberries—fresh strawberries, strawberry preserves and strawberry pie.

The Complete Consideration of a Single Disease

Textbooks have long since made familiar the logical sequence: *definition, etiology, pathology, epidemiology, symptoms, diagnosis, differential diagnosis, prognosis, prophylaxis* and *treatment*. Occasionally a single disease may be fully and completely considered under all these headings. Such a study may be made in the preparation of textbook material or of an article to be included in a system of medicine. Again, the sudden outbreak in epidemic form of an unusual illness or even of some common disease may make it worthwhile to review the subject completely for periodical publication. Ordinarily the writer will find it satisfactory to confine himself to the single phase of the disease which he wishes to discuss and on which he has something new to offer. This caution may seem unnecessary, but many manuscripts are received in which the reporting of a single new observation has been made an occasion to repeat much material that is easily available in the ordinary textbook.

The Monograph

A monograph is a special treatise on a single subject. Usually after an author has made an extensive series of investigations on some topic, he desires to present all the material in a single publication. In preparing a monograph, he will do well to outline all the material in order to avoid duplication. Only the special periodicals publish monographs, and because of their character the author may be asked to bear a portion of the expense.

SUMMARY AND CONCLUSIONS

The summary—a brief abstract of the article—may appear at the beginning or at the close. Not every article should be summarized. Those of more than average length (more than 1,500 words), those which involve much description of detail and technic and those which aim at a complete survey of literature on the particular subject demand a summary. A brief digest of a long article in the introductory paragraph often will stimulate someone to read the article who otherwise would not.

The summary should recapitulate observations reported or repeat statements of fact. The writer should not say simply that certain phases of a subject are discussed or that a certain type of case is reported. Such a summary wastes space without giving additional information or emphasizing significant facts. Manuscript editors usually will delete sentences offered as a summary which are without importance in emphasizing the material in the article itself.

The conclusions—the deductions drawn from the cases presented, the experiments or other facts set forth— appear at the close. Conclusions are of special value, particularly since they lead to wider abstracting. Conclusions are "fat" for abstracters and for editors who are looking for fillers. If an author is anxious to have his conclusions reproduced by other journals, he should rigidly condense them, yet make them clearly reflect his premises and deductions.

Conclusions, which usually are more or less coordinate in structure and substance, frequently gain effectiveness by being numbered. Items in a summary or in a combination of summary and conclusions, however, as a rule should not be numbered, for they are not coordinate. In the following example the numbering is correct. Had all the paragraphs been numbered consecutively, the effect would be illogical and misleading.

> A series of 103 cases of various functional dermatoses and 7 cases of true eczema were studied. . . .
>
> Every patient was subjected to epidermal and dermal testing by means of patch tests and scratch tests performed with a standard set of 74 substances. . . .
>
> From the data obtained we believe that the following conclusions may be drawn:
>
> 1. Epidermal hypersensitivity as manifested by a positive reaction to a patch test is present in patients with eczema—dermatitis venenata as an unchanging reaction to the causative substance.
>
> 2. Epidermal hypersensitivity is rarely, if ever, present in patients with functional dermatoses.
>
> 3. Dermal hypersensitivity as manifested by a positive reaction to a scratch test is noted occasionally in patients with eczema, and the causative substance is frequently the cause of an accompanying hay fever or asthma.

The value of the summary and the conclusions is appreciated less by the average writer than by the average reader. The busy physician looks at the title to see whether the subject interests him, glances at the subheads to see the phases considered and then turns to the summary to get the gist of the article. If he finds that he is especially interested, he then reads the whole paper.

NOTES OF ACKNOWLEDGMENT

Expressions of gratitude to all the persons who have given assistance, advice or encouragement to an author in his work are without scientific value and therefore out of place in the pages of a scientific journal. They may, however, be included in the author's reprints. If a person has rendered service of major importance, his name should be included with those of the authors of the paper. If he is thought to deserve not quite so much prominence, a form such as the following may be used:

JOHN BROWN, M.D.
With the Assistance of James Jones, M.A.

If only a slight contribution has been made a note may be included (at the beginning or at the end of the article or as a footnote) which gives a simple statement of the service rendered; for instance, "Dr. ———— prepared the photographs."

A statement that another physician gave "advice," "encouragement" or "inspiration" is not sufficiently specific to be included. The definite part of the work which he performed should be mentioned.

QUOTED MATERIAL

When material is quoted from the work of another author, the laws governing copyrights require that permission be secured from the copyright holder and courtesy would suggest that this also be from the author. An editor who accepts many papers each week cannot ask in each instance if written permission has been secured. The responsibility must rest with the author.

Material which is quoted should be quoted exactly, unless there are obvious typographic errors. Frequently when an author is preparing an article he copies essential statements with lead pencil. Later he uses the notes verbatim in his paper, forgetting that they may not have been copied accurately. A physician who wishes to use quotations should either have an accurate typewritten copy made of all material he may wish to quote when he consults the book or periodical or, if this is not feasible, should have the chosen passages rechecked when the final copy of his manuscript is being made.

Laboratory reports made by other physicians, personal communications and other material which has not been published elsewhere may, and should, be edited in the same style as that used for the rest of the paper. Such material usually is not written for publication and is not prepared as carefully as it would have been had the writer known it would appear in print under his name.

4
CONSTRUCTION OF THE MANUSCRIPT

IDEALLY, the framework of a paper should be outlined before writing is begun. This framework may include headings for short imaginary chapters, each chapter covering a subdivision of the subject. If the article is to be elaborate, each heading may be further subdivided. This will avoid the repetition of facts or ideas —a common fault. A suitable title, informative subheads, a clear summary and cogent conclusions represent the framework of a well-constructed paper.

THE TITLE

The title is more important than the average medical writer realizes. If an author wants his contribution to become a part of the literature on the subject, he must give it a name that will identify it and that is descriptive. Thousands of papers lie buried in medical literature because their titles did not designate the subjects. The title should be short, but inclusiveness should not be sacrificed for brevity. Often a long title may seem necessary, although usually brevity and clearness may be gained by the use of a main title and a subtitle. A title should consist of not more than 90 letters, counting spaces between words as letters.

Hardly anyone remembers such unwieldly titles as "Brain Tumor of Psychomotor Area, Causing Jacksonian and Generalized Convulsions, Visual Hallucinations: Somatic Operation; Recovery, Mental and Physical." With that title, why write a paper? Another unwieldly example: "Erythromelalgia: Report of a Case

Presenting Peripheral Vasomotor Disturbances in the Hands and Feet for Twelve Years, Reaching a Climax in Eight Years, with Recovery Following Treatment by Adrenal Substance." These two examples are taken from published papers. The following was the original title of a paper that was submitted for publication. "To Obtain Graphs Showing the Rapidity and Degree of Decrease in Temperature in the Eye and Orbit Produced by the External Application of a Given Degree of Cold over a Given Area for a Given Time, and a Numerical Expression, at Least Approximate, of the Relation of These Variables to Each Other." What could an indexer or cataloguer do with such a title? This title should be rewritten thus: "Coefficient of Thermal Conductivity of Eye and Orbit Measured with Application of Cold."

Ambiguity

Misleading titles should be avoided. "A New Chloroform Danger" was the caption of another manuscript. In looking up references to the literature on the dangers of anesthesia a physician would have been attracted by the title, and after laboriously searching for the article he would have discovered that he had been misled. The title became "Danger in Similarity of Ether and Chloroform Containers," which stated the subject of the communication. First impressions are lasting; a catchy title catches readers. The title ought to be carefully thought out and should give a clear indication of what is to come.

The following titles, taken from papers published in medical periodicals, are examples of the ambiguous types which cause distress to those responsible for indexing medical literature:

Foci of Infections Above Collar Bone and Importance of Their Early Recognition
Borderline Cases
"Ideas in" Syphilology
Odd Experience of a Young Practitioner
The Emergency Abdomen
The Abused Cervix

Idle Thoughts on Medical Education
Render unto Caesar
Macedonian Call
School Follicles
Curing, from Yon to Hither
Clinical Observations
Suggestions
Sepelire Malum Resuscitare Bonum
Some Stomachs I Have Met

The Subtitle

If it is necessary to include much material in the title, it should be divided into a main title and a subtitle. For example, the title "A Precise and Simple Method for Counting of Blood Cells and Bacteria Without a Special Chamber" became "Counting of Blood Cells and Bacteria," with the subtitle "A Precise and Simple Method Without a Special Chamber." Disturbances of Conditioned Reflexes Observed in Study of Functional Changes in the Brain of the Dog After Removal of the Cerebral Blood Supply, in This Case by Ligation of the Arteries Supplying It" might be expressed as a main title, "Functional Changes in the Brain of the Dog After Reduction of Its Blood Supply," and a subtitle, "Disturbances of Conditioned Reflexes After Ligation of Arteries."

The following are some examples of poor original titles and the way in which they were improved:

THREE HUNDRED AND THIRTY LOW, CERVICAL CESAREAN SECTIONS (LAPAROTRACHELOTOMIES) WITH TWO DEATHS

was changed to

LOW, OR CERVICAL, CESAREAN SECTION (LAPAROTRACHELOTOMY)
THREE HUNDRED AND THIRTY OPERATIONS, WITH TWO DEATHS

A CASE OF DERMATITIS GANGRENOSA INFANTUM

was changed to

DERMATITIS GANGRENOSA INFANTUM
REPORT OF A CASE

STUDY OF A CASE OF ACNITIS, WITH PARTICULAR REFERENCE TO THE BACTERIOLOGIC FINDINGS

was changed to
ACNITIS, WITH PARTICULAR REFERENCE TO
THE BACTERIOLOGIC FINDINGS
REPORT OF A CASE

———

FURTHER STUDIES IN ECZEMA AND DERMATITIS
was changed to
ECZEMA AND DERMATITIS

———

SYNDROME OF AVELLIS, WITH A REPORT
OF THREE CASES
was changed to
SYNDROME OF AVELLIS
REPORT OF THREE CASES

———

BACTERIOLOGIC STUDIES IN ACUTE ENTERITIS
IN INFANTS AND YOUNG CHILDREN, INCLUD-
ING BACTERIOLOGIC METHODS, MORPHOL-
OGY AND CULTURAL CHARACTERISTICS
OF STREPTOCOCCUS MICRO-APOIKIA
AND CLINICAL STUDIES ON
FORTY-SIX PATIENTS
WITH ACUTE
ENTERITIS
was changed to
ACUTE ENTERITIS IN INFANTS AND IN
YOUNG CHILDREN
BACTERIOLOGIC, MORPHOLOGIC AND CULTURAL STUDIES OF
STREPTOCOCCUS MICRO-APOIKIA; CLINICAL STUDIES
ON FORTY-SIX PATIENTS

———

THE STUDY OF BRONCHIAL ASTHMA AND
ALLIED ALLERGIC DISORDERS UNDER
CONTROLLED CONDITIONS OF
ENVIRONMENT, TEMPERA-
TURE AND HUMIDITY.
A PRELIMINARY
REPORT

was changed to

BRONCHIAL ASTHMA AND ALLIED ALLERGIC DISORDERS

PRELIMINARY REPORT OF A STUDY UNDER CONTROLLED CONDITIONS OF ENVIRONMENT, TEMPERATURE AND HUMIDITY

THE AUTHOR'S NAME

Much unnecessary confusion arises in the indexing of medical literature because authors sign their names in different manners in different countries. In France and in Germany many writers sign only their surnames; others use only initials for the first name. Many authors in foreign publications sign the name at the close of the article.

The Italians sometimes write the given name last. The Spanish frequently follow the father's surname with the mother's maiden name, and it is difficult to tell which is the baptismal name and which the surname. For example, Dr. Remigio Salazar should be indexed as R. Salazar, under the S's, while Dr. Alvárez Sierra is Dr. Alvárez and Sierra is to be disregarded. Then again, for personal reasons some Spanish writers prefer to be known by the mother's family name; so Dr. Angel Pérez Martín is always called Dr. Martín and Dr. Gómez y Giocoechea, Dr. Giocoechea. Professor Santiago Ramón y Cajal signed himself Cajal, rather than Ramón. References to the works of these men, however, should be indexed under the father's surname, the name being listed, for instance, as Pérez-Martín, A.

Chinese names usually are written with the surname first and the name which corresponds to the Christian name second, in two words with a hyphen between them; for instance, Wu Lien-tech. Some write their names with the surname last but still hyphenate the given name, as Lien-tech Wu. Still others use only the initials, in which case the surname is always the last, as L. T. Wu. When the second name is not hyphenated, it is difficult to know which is the surname and which the given name. When there is only one word to the second name, the surname should always be written first, as Wu Hsien, when Wu is the family name. In a few instances there are two syllables in the surname as well as in the given name; then the first two should be the surname, as Ou-Yang Yu-shen.

Obviously, in consulting American and English literature, the Spanish-speaking physician is at a loss and is likely to refer to Dr. Oliver Wendell Holmes as Dr. Wendell. The American practice in recording literature, that of giving the last name first, followed by a comma and the given name, sometimes produces errors; thus Dr. Ruth Tunnicliff is mentioned frequently in foreign indexes as Dr. Tunnicliff Ruth, and Dr. Marion Van Slyke sometimes is referred to as Dr. Van S. Marion. A young author should decide early in his career the manner in which he wishes his name to appear and should not change thereafter. Sir William Osler always signed his communications "W. Osler." Obviously, if the name is a common one, such as Smith, Brown or Johnson, and only the first initial is signed by the author, identification for indexing purposes is not easy. It is advisable for authors whose names are not widely known to sign the full name or, in any event, to adopt a consistent form and to follow it regularly.

HEADINGS AND SUBHEADINGS

Headings and subheadings help the reader to find the points which interest him most. Center heads break up pages of solid type, which repel the eye, and they aid the author to present his subject logically. It is to be regretted that center heads are not used more commonly in medical and other scientific journals.

If the author has prepared his article systematically, he will have collected his material according to various phases of the subject. Thus he may have an introduction, bibliographic references arranged chronologically or by classes, case reports, protocols of experiments, a summary and conclusions. Obviously, these represent center headings under which may come still more detailed subheads. Subheadings may take additional work, but it is worthwhile; they make the article more attractive and thus more likely to be read. The author is more competent than the copy editor to furnish subheadings.

As the author plans his structure, he should bear in mind

that all material under one heading should belong to it and that if the subject is changed, another heading must be inserted.

TYPE

Use of Italics

Excessive use of italic type detracts from the simplicity of style desirable in scientific works. In the publications of the American Medical Association italics are used sparingly. They are permitted for emphasis of words or phrases only when the effect can be secured in no other way.

Greek Letters and Symbols

When Greek letters are used they should be carefully inserted in ink, using a pen with a sharp point. It is desirable to identify them for the typesetter, either by writing the name of each letter in full in the margin or by using an accepted code number. These are sometimes included in the handbooks supplied authors by certain publishers.

Mathematical and other symbols likewise should be identified in the margin. Minus signs should be clearly indicated, as they may be confused with hyphens; use one hyphen with space at both sides, but omit the space after the hyphen when the sign represents a negative quantity and is not an indication of subtraction. Write the plus sign in ink unless the symbol is available as such on the typewriter.

Every man who writes should know a little bit about printing. An author who does will know how to prepare his manuscripts properly. Not one in a hundred has such knowledge. Avoidable wastes add to the cost and are stupidities that printers should try to eliminate.

5
WORDS AND PHRASES

SOLECISMS

Attention is called to the following paragraphs regarding solecisms quoted from an editorial by William H. Woglom:

Due to. This expression is a problem. Fowler says that this expression is used by the illiterate as though it had passed, like "owing to," into a mere compound preposition, whereas "due," like ordinary participles and adjectives, must be attached to a noun and not to a notion extracted from a sentence. Webster's "New International Dictionary" defines "due" as: "owing . . . *(to* something) . . . as, his death was *due* to pneumonia; often erroneously used in the phrase *due to,* meaning 'because of,' modifying a verb in the manner of a compound preposition; as, he failed *due* to lack of study."

Hypothecate. This does not mean "to make a hypothesis," as some seem to think, but "to deposit as security."

Data. The word "data" is a plural noun. Never, *never,* never write "the data *is.*"

Blastogenic. This is coming into use to mean "giving rise to tumors," but it should not be so employed because it was established long ago to describe Weissmann's theory of blastogenesis. Accordingly, Dr. Esmond R. Long, Medical Editor of Webster's "New International Dictionary," was asked to suggest a substitute. Consultation with his fellow editors led to the decision that "blastogenic" is an erroneous compound of blastoma, and the word "blastomatogenic" was proposed.

Butter Yellow. This expression should not be used because it has been applied to four different compounds, hence is ambiguous. Furthermore, considerable anxiety already has been aroused among the lay public on account of the perfectly natural misapprehension that butter yellow is used to color butter. For these reasons the chemical rather than the popular name should be selected.

Procarcinogen. The term "procarcinogen" should not be used. Since "pro" in biochemistry denotes a precursor, as in "prothrombin," the preferred word is "cocarcinogen," and "procarcinogen" will be reserved until such time as the precursors of naturally occurring carcinogens may be discoverd.

Medical Jargon

Many words with unusual meanings that are not recognized even by medical dictionaries have found their way into medical vocabularies. Such writings may be characterized as medical jargon or medical slang. When these words appear in medical manuscripts or in medical conversation, they are unintelligible to other scientists, particularly to those of foreign countries, since they are not translatable. They are the mark of the careless and uncultured person.

A number of these terms are given here, with the correct words following.

Jargon	*Correct Term*
acute abdomen	acute condition within the abdomen
alcoholic (as noun)	alcoholic addict, person with alcoholism
Ammon's horn	cornu ammonis
cardiac, cardiac patient	patient with cardiac disease
cardiac diet	diet for patients with cardiac disease
chronic appendix	chronic appendicitis
chronic ear	chronic otitis
diabetic (as noun)	person with diabetes
epileptic (as noun)	person with epilepsy
flu	influenza
jugular ligation	ligation of the jugular vein
lues, luetic	syphilis, syphilitic
milligrams per cent	milligrams per hundred grams [or] other unit
multip.	multipara
neisserian disease	gonorrhea
organ or structure is negative	organ or structure is normal
oviducts	fallopian tubes
pathology (in concrete sense)	pathologic change, disease
positive serology	positive serologic tests for syphilis
primip.	primipara
prostatic (as noun)	patient with hypertrophy, inflammation or some other disturbance of the prostate gland
right upper lobe	upper lobe of the right lung
serology	changes in the blood or serologic reactions of the blood or the spinal fluid

Jargon	Correct Term
specific	syphilitic, when that is meant
specific stomach	syphilis of the stomach
spinal fluid dynamics	dynamic pressure of spinal fluid
surgical (or operative) interference	surgical (or operative) intervention
subtotal gastrectomy	partial gastrectomy
suspicious of	suggestive of
syphilitic (as noun)	person with syphilis
taboparesis	the tabetic form of dementia paralytica
upper abdomen	upper part of the abdomen
upper respiratory infection	infection of the respiratory tract
urine contained 4 plus albumin	urine gave a 4 plus reaction for albumin [or] urine contained albumin (4 plus)

Certain forms of phraseology become established in medical discussions so that they are easily recognized by the physician but are ludicrous when written. Physicians frequently say that a patient was placed "on cannabis," "on hydrotherapy" or "on a diet." Probably most grammarians would sanction the last of these three phrases but would hesitate to approve the statement that the patient was "placed on cannabis." In such instances it is better for the writer to state that cannabis was prescribed in a certain dose, to be administered at certain periods in a certain manner. A physician may say, "I have had no experience with starvation in epilepsy." Obviously he means that he has not tried the treatment of epilepsy by starvation of the patient. He will say, "I have had little experience with pneumothorax in tuberculosis," meaning that he has not attempted the use of this method in any case of tuberculosis which has come to his attention.

Trite Usage

Many a competent journalist has urged reporters to use words that say exactly what is meant and to avoid the diction that has become trite by overusage. A good reporter never says "Smith sustained an injury"; he says "Smith was injured." He never writes that people were "joined in the holy bonds of matrimony"; he says "they were married." It is unnecessary to say of a well-known man that he is "well known" and, in any event, "widely known" is better than "well known." A dog is just a dog and not a "canine," exactly as a cow is a cow and not a "bovine." People begin various processes; they seldom "inaugurate" or "initiate" these affairs. A patient lives in Portland; he is not "located" in Portland. The body of a dead man is his "body" and not his "remains." Far too many sentences begin with the words "It is" and "There is."

Case

A case is an instance of disease, the totality of the symptoms and of the pathologic and other conditions; a patient is the human being afflicted. One continually finds in medical manuscripts such sentences as "The case had a fever," "Thirty cases were admitted to the hospital" and "The case was operated on." In the publications of the American Medical Association such usages are banned.

A less-obvious confusion exists in the employment of "case" to designate the condition. While from the definitions of the word given in dictionaries it might be used in the narrow sense of an attack of a disease, in which event it might be considered as the condition itself, such usage is likely to lead to constant shifting of the point of view, even within sentences or paragraphs. One might write, for instance, "In the acute case the patient was admitted to the hospital." Obviously, a case which is acute includes only the actual disease and its symptoms, while a case in which admission to the hospital is made and records are kept must include far more—all the attendant circumstances. Thus the word would be used in two senses in the same sentence. To avoid such inconsistency, proper medical writing restricts the use of "case" to its broader meaning, as indicated in the preceding paragraph—an instance of disease, the totality of what is known about the patient, his condition and all the circumstances. Moreover, the concrete subjects with which one is dealing are the patient and his condition, and writing will be simplified and vivified if one refers to them specifically rather than to the abstract "case".

Use of Abstract Words in a Concrete Sense

"A malignancy was removed," "The cytology was normal" and similar statements are found frequently in manuscripts. For many years my policy has been to avoid the use of abstract words in a concrete sense. The suffix "ology," for instance, according to Webster, means "a science or branch of knowledge"; and to use a word with that ending to describe a tumor or a specific change in the tissue is illogical and inconsistent with the principles of good choice of words. "There was no pathology" is an outrageous sentence. One would not dream of saying "There was no ophthalmology," for instance. The use of "etiology" as a synonym for "cause" is a similar common abuse of the language. Again, "etiology" is a broad term meaning the science or study of the causes of disease.

The following incorrect and correct sentences illustrate the principles that should be followed in the preparation and in the editing of manuscripts.

Incorrect	Correct
The growth proved not to be a malignancy.	The tumor was not malignant.
	The malignancy of the growth was not established.
There was no pathology.	A pathologic condition was not found.
	The pathology[1] of syphilis is worthy of much study.
The morphology of the tissue was that of sarcoma.	The structure of the growth showed it to be a sarcoma.
The histology of the lesion was studied.	The lesion was examined histologically (or microscopically).
The cytology was normal.	The cells (or cell count or whatever specific features were noted) were normal.
The patient presented a severe symptomatology.	The patient had severe symptoms.
	A knowledge of symptomatology aids the physician in diagnosis.
	The symptomatology of tuberculosis is varied.[2]
The etiology of the anemia shown by this patient was not known.	In this case the cause of the anemia was not determined.
	The etiology[3] of some diseases is still vague.

Incorrect	Correct
Microscopy showed the changes to be well advanced.	Microscopic examination revealed the nature of the tumor.
Bronchoscopy was performed immediately.	A bronchoscopic examination was performed immediately.
	Treatment with the bronchoscope relieved the patient.
	The development of bronchoscopy has aided the physician greatly.
Ventriculography showed normal filling.	A ventriculogram was made on several occasions.
	Encephalography should be understood by every neurologist.
Surgery seemed the only possible treatment for that patient.	Surgical intervention was considered but was postponed.
	(Title) Surgery of the Gallbladder.[4]

Dosage and Dose

"Dosage" means the administration of medicine in regular doses or the determination and regulation of the proper doses. The amount of a medicament to be administered at one time is correctly termed the "dose." Such expressions as "administered in small dosage" or "dosage of 3 drops" are redundant and should be avoided, and the shorter and more concrete word "dose" should be employed.

Inject

The transitive verb "inject" means (1) to introduce a substance into or (2) to distend or fill with fluid by injection. It is therefore incorrect to speak of "injecting a patient with arsphenamine" or of "injecting a rabbit with virus." One "gives the patient

---

[1] "Pathology" here means the part of the science of pathology that deals with syphilis.

[2] "Symptomatology" here refers to the entire complex of symptoms known to be associated with tuberculosis.

[3] "Etiology" here means the theories of the causation of the disease. "Causation," however, would be better.

[4] "Surgery" may be used in an instance such as this if the author wants to emphasize that he is dealing with the part of the entire field of surgery that concerns the gallbladder. Usually, however, "Surgical Intervention on the Gallbladder" is adequate.

an injection" and "injects the virus into the rabbit" or "inoculates the rabbit with the virus." It is permissible, however, to say that one "injects the bronchi" or "injects the blood vessels of a cadaver" when one actually fills the structures with a contrast medium.

Temperature and Fever, and Analogous Expressions

To say that a patient had "no temperature" is incorrect. "No fever" or "no elevation of temperature" may be used, although it is perhaps better to say that the temperature is "normal" or "higher than normal" or "subnormal." Better still, if the temperature is abnormal, it should be given in terms of the Fahrenheit or centigrade scale. It is, moreover, incorrect to say that a patient had a "fever of 102° F"; "temperature" rather than "fever" should be used.

An analogous faulty usage occurs frequently with other words. "Leukocytosis," for instance, means the *presence* of an abnormally large number of white cells in the blood. It is undesirable, therefore, to speak of "leukocytosis of 15,000" instead of "a leukocyte count of 15,000." If an author wishes to emphasize the abnormal condition by the use of the word "leukocytosis," he may say that "leukocytosis was present (15,000 cells)" or that "there was leukocytosis, the white cell count being 15,000."

The Associated Press issued a bulletin calling attention to words frequently confused in newspapers. Here are some examples. Do not write, "Data is"; "actions" for "acts"; "dangerous condition" for "serious condition"; "from whence"; "the board are"; "different than"; "address" for "speech"; "filled to capacity"; "love" for "like"; "wonderful" when it is not; "enjoyed by all present"; "Jackson Robinson, son of Mr. and Mrs. James Robinson, and who"; "A car, standing beside the curb, and which"; "exotic" when it isn't; "drowned while swimming"; "automobile turned turtle," which only means to sink like a turtle; "partially" for "partly" destroyed; "replica" when it is not. Do write "Folies" not "Follies" Bergere; "du Pont" not "Dupont"; "Newnan, Ga." not "Newman, Ga."; and "widows" not "wives" as survivors of husbands.

Similarly, manuscripts frequently contain such expressions as "The glycemia increased from 90 to 125 mg per hundred cubic centimeters" and "There was hyperglycemia of 150 mg." These ideas would be expressed better as "The sugar content of the blood increased from 90 to 125 mg," "The sugar content was high, 150 mg per hundred cubic centimeters" or "There was hyperglycemia, the sugar content being 150 mg."

Cystoscope, Obstetricate, Explore, Refract

The following sentence appeared in a manuscript submitted for publication:

> It was decided that the patient should be explored with the expectation of finding an acute appendix.

Such a decision once made, the surgeon did not hesitate; he explored his patient. Another surgeon was not so courageous. He said,

> We have contemplated having some of our inoperable cases collapsed by thoracoplasty, but have delayed.

And another physician, finding the English language rather inadequate for his purpose, perpetrated this monstrosity:

> In a case in which I obstetricated at birth . . .

Such use of transitive verbs with illogical objects has no justification in the laws of grammar or in the usage of persons of even ordinary education. Even less justification exists for using ordinary common nouns as verbs which do not exist. Astronomers never telescope the sky; bacteriologists never microscope their slides; but urologists do not hesitate to cystoscope their patients. Far worse, however, is the conversion of proper names of scientists into verbs describing procedures that they have evolved or discovered. The bacteriologist who would not microscope his slides will "Schick" one patient and "Wassermann" another.

Use of Adjectives as Nouns

Some words, such as "juveniles," "adolescents," "adults" and "convalescents," which originally were pure adjectives and are still adjectival in form, have come to be accepted as nouns. In most instances, however, it is well to avoid the use of an adjective as a substantive, from the standpoint both of linguistic purity and of accuracy in medical terminology. "Sphenoid" and "ethmoid" are now listed in medical dictionaries as nouns designating the respective bones; their use in a similar way to indicate the sinuses, however, is not sanctioned and is misleading to the reader, who frequently is unable to determine which structure is meant. Neurologists frequently speak of "the sympathetic" or "the sympathetics." How much more informative it would be if in each instance some specific phrase, such as "the sympathetic nervous system," "the sympathetic nerve supply of the area," "sympathetic nerve fibers" or "the cervical portion of the sympathetic trunk," were supplied! Use of the adjectives designating arteries, veins, nerves and muscles as substantives may cause a reader to puzzle, for instance, over whether an artery, a vein or a nerve is meant when an author speaks of "the iliac" or "the peroneal."

"The former" or "the latter" refers to one of two specific things just mentioned and therefore may be considered as having a specific antecedent, making insertion of a noun in each instance unnecessary. In the case of "the foregoing" and "the following," however, the exact thing referred to may not be as clear as it should be in scientific writing, so usually it is better to supply the noun which the author has in mind, as "the foregoing list" or "the following formula."

Some terms are so frequently used in various phases of medical practice that they become recognized as in good usage. For instance, the industrial physician has employed the following terms so frequently that their use is permissible:

accident proneness labor union
case finding occupational hazard examination
employee morale plant supervision
employee union union grievance
health audit work stoppage
health examination

In other phases of medical practice, other combinations have also been so frequently used as to be recognized as good form. Here are some examples:

blood cultures
blood plasma
brain damage
brain injury
cataract extraction
lid margin

lower back pain
skin flap
skin reaction
skull fracture
urinary tract infection

Adjectives Modifying a Word Other Than the One Qualified

Such expressions as "the right chest" and "the upper abdomen" are commonly used. Since there is only one of each of these structures and the adjective really modifies an understood "side" or "part," the phrases should be expanded to "right side of the chest" or "upper portion of the abdomen" or some equally accurate designation.

A similar misuse of adjectives occurs in such phrases as "upper respiratory infection," which means, and should be expressed as, "infection of the upper part of the respiratory tract." Other undesirable phrases of this type are the following:

right heart	for	right side of the heart (specify right ventricle or right auricle)
cardiac diet	for	diet for patients with cardiac disease
jugular ligation	for	ligation of the jugular vein
facial paralysis	for	paralysis of the facial nerve, when that is meant
left lower lobe	for	lower lobe of the left lung

Further illustrations are included in the list of examples of medical jargon on pages 47 and 48.

Group and Type

A favorite of many physicians is the word "group." An author may divide his patients into "groups" on the basis of age, again on the basis of the type of disease presented and finally on the basis of the results obtained. In many instances confusion may be avoided by using other terms, such as "series" and "subgroup," to distinguish the divisions concerned.

The use of "group" in the sense of "type," however, as in the phrase "this group of sarcoma," should be avoided not only because of vagueness but also because of inaccuracy. Funk and Wagnalls' *New College Standard Dictionary* gives eight definitions of "group" and Webster gives twelve; but none of them justifies this use of the word. Frequently an author says after a sentence has been questioned that he means a group of cases of a particular type of tumor, but he did not bring this out in the manuscript. The following examples of correct usage should be considered carefully:

> In the first group of cases sarcoma of the spindle-cell type occurred.
> This type of growth belongs to the lymphoblastoma group (that is, a group of several related structures all of which are lymphoblastomas).
> The type of lymphoblastoma under consideration is interesting.

Carelessness in writing and in organization of material is evident when, for instance, an author defines three groups of *cases,* numbered 1, 2 and 3, and then proceeds to speak of "the *patients* of group 1" or "the *tumors* of group 3."

Indefinite Article Before the Name of a Condition

Idiom requires that one say "The boy had an eruption." "The patient had anemia," however, is preferable to "The patient had an anemia," for both clarity and brevity. With the names of most conditions which are definite entities, "a" or "an" may be omitted to advantage.

The plural forms of names of conditions, such as "anemias" and "toxemias," usually should not be employed in the sense of instances of the condition but should be reserved to designate types of the condition. "The anemias that I have observed" might mean either "the forms of anemia that I have observed" or "the cases of anemia that I have observed." If the latter is meant, the fact is brought out by insertion of "cases of" or "instances of."

Operate

A flagrant disregard of the rules of grammar is found in the deplorable misuse of the verb "operate." "Operate" is both a transitive and an intransitive verb, and its usage in the two forms is clearly defined in even the most elementary grammar. "Operate" means, and is synonymous with, "work." The terms nearly always may be used interchangeably. The surgeon who would hesitate to say "I worked this patient" says unblushingly "I operated this patient." This solecism is limited to the medical profession. It is also limited to this country. American surgeons who justify themselves by saying that general usage makes correct usage should realize that "operate" is a word in general use wherever the English language is spoken, and that members of other professions and trades use it correctly. Even if this misuse of the verb "operate" were not limited to medicine, good usage is the usage not of the careless minority but of the educated majority. The pity of it is that some teachers in medical schools—professors of surgery—instead of setting an example to their students in the proper use of this verb, are responsible for the spread of its improper use.

Milligrams Per Cent

Results of chemical determinations frequently are expressed as "milligrams per cent" or "grams per cent." This means literally "milligrams (or grams) per hundred milligrams (or grams)," which in most instances is not the information that the author wishes to convey. To insure accuracy a writer should specify the unit used, such as "milligrams per hundred cubic centimeters" or "milligrams per hundred grams." If a number of values are given close together in a section or in a short paper, it usually is sufficient to supply "per hundred cubic centimeters" the first time the phrase appears and to use merely "milligrams" (not "milligrams per cent") thereafter.

Findings and Found

An autopsy or a histologic examination of tissue is in most instances a systematic study of organs and tissues for the purpose of learning what changes, if any, have taken place. Preferably therefore, speak of the conditions "observed," "seen" or "noted" rather than of those "found," and refer to "observations" rather than to "findings." In the publications of the American Medical Association Press this distinction is observed, except perhaps in instances in which a search for a specific element is being made and the element is therefore actually found, as is frequently true in microscopic studies of blood and of cultures.

The word "findings" is, in general, overworked. If an author will look over a paper to see how often he has mentioned "findings" and in how many instances something more specific could have been substituted, he frequently will be surprised and will be able to make his report more informative.

Histologic and Histopathologic

Some writers have acquired a habit of using "histopathologic" to the exclusion of the briefer word "histologic." There may be instances in which the idea of disease or of a relation to the science of pathology that is expressed by "-patho-" gives additional information. If it is known, however, that the tissues examined are from a tumor or are part of a body under the influence of a general disease," "histologic examination" or "the changes observed histologically" is adequate.

Developed

According to the *Pocket Oxford Dictionary,* the verb "develop" means "bring or come from a latent or rudimentary or immature state to visibility or activity or greater elaboration or size or completeness." Other dictionaries agree. It is obviously incorrect, therefore, to say that a patient "developed a tumor," for he did not bring it into being. When "develop" is used with reference to the origin of disease, it must be employed in its intransitive sense, as in the sentence: "The disease developed in this patient when he was six years old."

Biopsy

The term "biopsy" is variously defined by dictionaries. Many physicians employ the word to cover both the surgical removal of a specimen from the living subject and its examination under the microscope. I believe it is best to adopt this broader sense which includes the whole procedure. To speak of "biopsy examination" is redundant.

VAGUE AND INACCURATE TERMS

Ambiguous Pronouns

Confusion is caused by careless use of pronouns. It often is impossible to tell when an author is referring to himself and when to some other person or persons. He may refer to himself in one place as "the writer," in another as "I" and in still another as "we." He may then use the pronoun "we" with reference to the medical profession or to people in general. The use of the first person singular ("I" or "me") is usually the clearest and most satisfactory usage.

In a supplement to the *Lancet*[5] it was stated:

> The first person singular—the naked *I*—is no longer thought immodest. Elaborate garments such as *we* and *the author* do not disguise a writer's identity unless they also disguise his meaning; and medicine has no need of such aids to ambiguity.

In the past, when the individual physician undertook the complete medical care of his patient, the editorial *we* was much more widely used. Today, the personal physician in a teaching or general hospital needs auxiliary personnel and services to meet the standards of modern care. In reporting a case the distinction between *I* and *we* may be essential for accurate communication.

Many important scientific discoveries, which might now be attributed to serendipity, were the result of one investigator's observations. Now scientists work in teams which often represent many disciplines.

Multiple Authors. At one period in the rise of modern medicine a writer would name his associates in a note of thanks appended to the research report. Today, the names of all who have made a significant contribution to the project are listed among the authors responsible for the published results. In addition, the report acknowledges the support of various philanthropies, voluntary foundations and government agencies. Mention is made of the institution in which the work was done, as well as the hospital or laboratory that provided the necessary personnel and equipment.

Under the system that once prevailed in most universities, the department head took responsibility for the research conducted in his division. In most foreign universities, his name invariably appeared on every manuscript coming out of the department. Research begun under this professor's direction was sometimes car-

---
[5] On writing for the *Lancet. Lancet,* Jan. 2, 1937, supp., p. i.

ried on for months in his absence, yet the published work included his name.

When the plural pronoun was habitually used, readers took for granted that not only the individual physician but also the staff of his hospital or research institute agreed to take responsibility for the publication. This was not always the case. In fact, instances have occurred in which investigators of equal rank and authority have expressed disagreement, a fact that was not recorded in the report itself. In such cases, the use of *we* was obviously misleading.

According to Fowler's *Modern English Usage*, the pronoun "we" may be used in an editorial and generic sense. However, says Fowler, "Writers of books and articles should not use we in circumstances where the collective anonymity of the editorial of a newspaper is out of place." An author should not use *we* instead of *I* in expressing a personal preference, nor should he hide awkwardly behind the cloak of "the present writer."

Modern authors, Fowler points out, are bolder than was formerly fashionable in the use of *I*. Perhaps out of misplaced modesty, however, many scientists avoid the personal pronoun entirely. These writers describe their experiments in the passive voice—*Such-and-such a thing was done.* "This trick," as Fowler says, "becomes wearisome by repetition, and makes the reader long for the author to break the monotony by saying boldly, 'I did *such-and-such a thing.*'"

When an author is reporting work done in conjunction with others, it is proper for him to use the prononun "we," provided he states who are represented by the "we," so that the reader will not be confused. When reference is made to one of two or three joint authors, the correct form is "one of us," with either the initials or the name in parentheses if the authors wish it.

The use of "the writer" or "the author" when the author of the paper means himself often makes it difficult to tell whether the author of the paper or another author just referred to is meant. Such usage is not permitted in most periodicals published by established medical publishers. In impartial reviews of the literature, in which the author is abstracting earlier papers by himself, alone or in collaboration with others, as impersonally as reports by other physicians, it is permissible for him to say "Jones and Brown reported . . . " instead of "Brown and I reported . . . " if awkwardness is avoided by use of this form.

As an example of the difficulty occasioned by improper use of the word "we," the following incident is cited: An author used the plural pronoun all through his paper. One sentence originally read

> Feeling as we do, we have ceased to employ it unless for some exceptional reason.

This was changed to

> The hospital staff has ceased to use radium unless for some exceptional reason.

The author, in going over his proof, made the sentence read

> Personally, we have ceased to use radium unless for some exceptional reason.

The manuscript editor, anticipating trouble, spoke about this when the proof was returned and suggested that the statement might read:

> Radium is no longer used in the clinics at the New York Post-Graduate Medical School and Hospital.

This suggestion was not put into type but was submitted to the author for his approval with a letter relative to the use of the plural pronoun, saying:

> As you will notice, we have made a *suggestion* on the last galley to obviate the use of the plural pronoun.

He apparently took offense at this suggestion for modifying the sentence, for in his letter returning the proof he said:

> I refer particularly to the end of the article where you have made a decided change in the wording. You have also caused me to state what is not correct (the fourth paragraph from the end) when you substitute "is no longer used in the clinics at the Post-Graduate Hospital."

The author finally changed the sentence to read:

> Personally, I have ceased to use radium . .

The use of the pronoun "you" when physicians in general or people in general are meant is also confusing.

In reports of meetings of societies "we" and "you" may be used to refer to the members.

Overworked Phrases

Certain locutions are likely to become established as a part of the vocabulary of the physician. Such phrases as "the examination revealed," "the microscope showed," "significant observation," "points out," "unexplored fields," "throws light," "symptom complex," "so-called," "suffered from the disease" (meaning "had"), "complains of the disease" and "interesting and instructive" are so frequently used by authors that they are likely to pass over them even after five or six readings of their manuscripts. A special revision should be planned to eliminate overworked phrases.

Superlatives—Very, Quite, Marked, Great

Physicians and scientists frequently seem to find difficulty in expressing comparative size or comparative degrees of severity of illness; hence such words as "very," "quite," "marked" and "great" are used to excess.

The use of "very" was discussed by Franklin P. Adams in the New York *Tribune*. He said:

> Years ago this Pisa of Puristics, buttressed by Mr. Gelett Burgess, offered a prize for an instance of the adverbial use of "very" that made the qualified word stronger. As we recall it, "Very good, Eddie" and "the Very Reverend Somebody" were the only offerings. The use of "very" in speaking or writing is a confession of verbal poverty and mental indolence.

The true meaning of "quite" is "completely." The use of the word in the sense of "considerably" is designated as colloquial (United States) in the *Pocket Oxford Dictionary* and in the *Standard Dictionary* and as loose or erroneous by Webster. Moreover, "The skin was quite red" tells the reader no more than does "The skin was red."

When "quite" (except in its strictly correct sense) or "very" appears in an article accepted for publication in one of the periodicals of the American Medical Association, the word usually is deleted by the manuscript editors.

In an editorial in the *Archives of Dermatology and Syphilology*,[6] Dr. William Allen Pusey, then and for many years its editor, presented the following discussion of the use of the word "marked":

> The too frequent use of the participial adjectives "marked" or "pronounced," when the writer means great, large, distinct, appreciable, moderate, considerable, extreme, intense or some other quality that he could easily, with a little thought, express accurately by means of a descriptive word, is perhaps the most frequent fault. "Marked" used in this indefinite sense was found four times in two short consecutive paragraphs in a manuscript written by an academic graduate of one of our famous colleges. The adverb "quite" is used in the same way; sometimes it is used as a diminutive adverb, as "quite frequently" for "occasionally," or to express all degrees of qualification from slightly to completely: "His mentality was quite low" for "His mentality was extremely low." The great objection to the loose use of such words as "marked" and "quite" is that the words when so used do not indicate accurately what qualifications the writer means.

On this subject Charles A. Mercier[7] wrote:

> It is to be regretted that we have never adopted the admirable proposal of Dean Swift, to keep all adjectives under lock and key, and issue them to writers only on payment of a heavy fee. Certain words are so shockingly overworked by medical writers as to call loudly for a Society for the Prevention of Cruelty to Adjectives. It would be invidious to quote from any individual writer to illustrate a vice so generally prevalent, and therefore I will disguise the reference by altering the disease; but mutatis mutandis, I recently read in your columns an account that ran much as follows: A marked erythema was followed by a marked ulceration, with a markedly sinuous edge, which spread with marked rapidity, and developed a marked discharge, having a markedly purulent character, increased to a markedly large size and was accompanied by a marked enlargement of the lymphatic glands. Treatment brought about a marked improvement with marked rapidity, and the ulcer healed, leaving a markedly thickened scar, which became the seat of marked keloid.

---

[6]Editorial: The careless writing of medical authors. *Arch. Dermat. Syph.*, 3:421, April 1921.

[7]Mercier, Charles A.: How medical writings may be given a marked development, Brit. M. J. 1:768 (May 20) 1916.

Above and Below

In preparing copy for publication it is well to avoid the use of the words "above" and "below," for one cannot know just where a passage will come on the printed page. The paragraph referred to as "above" may fall at the bottom of one page, and the one in which it is mentioned, at the top of another. The difficulty may be avoided by use of such a term as "mentioned," "previously mentioned" or "aforementioned," or by referring to the heading or subheading of the section in which the statement cited appears.

Et Cetera

"Et cetera" or "etc." should not be used in scientific articles, since the term conveys little if any idea of what was in the mind of the person who used it, and the manuscript editor usually is not able to substitute anything more specific. When "etc." follows "such as" or "for instance," it is superfluous.

Bilious

There was a time when anyone who was a little peaked and whose gastrointestinal tract was somewhat upset was characterized as "bilious." The term is a complete misnomer, since it does not refer to any actual disease. Scientific physicians have discarded it entirely.

Eczema

To the average layman, any disease of the skin is "eczema." Unfortunately, dermatologists themselves have fought over the term for many years. The word "eczema" refers to a certain type of reaction in the skin, as do the terms "urticaria," "erythema multiforme" and "erythema nodosum." The latter are definite types of reaction, due to numerous causes or often to unknown causes. An abundance of dermatologic papers have been concerned with the nature of eczema or eczematous types of eruption.

Neurasthenia, Psychasthenia and Hysteria

These terms are commonly used by the layman, together with "nervous breakdown," to describe any temperamental or mental disturbance. To the physician, they should indicate definite conditions.

Strain and Sprain

Some physicians refer to any disturbance in a muscle or a ligament as a strain, when in reality it is sometimes a sprain. These terms are ambiguous, since the exact condition constitutes a rupture of the tissues or perhaps a dislocation. The terms "strain" and "sprain" seems to be without exact significance.

Infection vs. Inflammation

When the body is invaded by bacteria, it is infected. When any portion of the body suffers irritation from any cause, bacterial or otherwise, it responds by becoming red, swollen and hot; this reaction is inflammation. The two terms are sometimes used interchangeably without any concept as to their actual meaning.

Rheumatism

The use of this word as a designation for any pain is not justified. It is misused particularly with reference to the disease known as arthritis, which is inflammation of a joint.

Asthma

The term "asthma" commonly is used to designate any disease in which there is shortness of breath. Actually, shortness of breath may result from one of many causes, including a disease known as bronchial asthma. The correct term for shortness of breath is "dyspnea."

PREFERRED USAGES

Among other usages which frequently appear in medical writings and which, while not incorrect, in some instances are susceptible of improvement are the following:

Word or Phrase	Preferred Usage
adrenalin	epinephrine
affection (except in the special neurologic sense)	disease

66 Medical Writing

Word or Phrase	Preferred Usage
agranulocytosis	granulocytopenia
all of	all
cane sugar	sucrose
carbon dioxide snow	solid carbon dioxide
casualty	wounded person
colored	Negro
cure (meaning treatment)	treatment (these words are not interchangeable)
deep roentgen therapy	high voltage roentgen therapy
doctor	physician
enteric fever	typhoid
functionating	functioning
general paresis, general paralysis, paretic dementia	dementia paralytica
Grave's disease, Basedow's disease	exophthalmic goiter
gut, guts*	intestine, intestines
Hebrew, Israelite	Jew, Jewish
hemeralopia	day blindness
humans	human beings, man
hyphema	hyphemia (indicating hemorrhage of the eye)
hypodermatic	hypodermic
in extremis	moribund, dying
individual	person
insanity	mental disease
leukocytic count	leukocyte count
lymph gland	lymph node
male, female	boy or man, girl or woman
medical men, men	physicians (or dermatologists, neurologists or some other specialists)
microphotograph	photomicrograph
milk sugar	lactose
mongolian, mongoloid (as noun)	person with mongolism
nyctalopia	night blindness
pediatrist	pediatrician
physiotherapist	physical therapist or physiatrist
physiotherapy	physical therapy
polynuclear (when referring to leukocytes)	polymorphonuclear
proven (archaic)	proved
remarks (in heading)	comment, observations

*"Gut" is used in embryology.

Word or Phrase	Preferred Usage
round-celled tumor	round cell tumor
sacrificed	killed
Scharlach R	scarlet red
skiagram	roentgenogram
spotted fever	specific disease meant, such as typhus, cerebrospinal meningitis or Rocky Mountain spotted fever
suprarenal	adrenal
therapeutist	therapist
treponeme	spirochete
tumor mass	tumor
ultraviolet light	ultraviolet rays
x-ray picture	roentgenogram

Foreign Phrases

From the time when the physician was characterized by his ability to discourse fluently in Latin, certain Latin phrases have filtered into medical discussions with a frequency that resembles the manner in which *Bacillus subtilis* may contaminate pure cultures of virulent germs. Terms frequently abused are: *pari passu, a priori, per se, in extenso, per os, in extremis* and *exitus lethalis.* How much better to say simply, "The patient died" than to indicate his passing to immortality by a Latin route.

Other foreign terms frequently used are *per contra, ad lib,* and *sub judice.* Such terms may be used but should be avoided when possible.

To doctors in different countries, the same medical terms may have opposite meanings. The term "nyctalopia" refers to night blindness in England and day blindness in France. Typhus means typhoid fever in Germany and France but suggests a different disease in English- and Spanish-speaking countries. Confusion in medical terminology is growing in such rapidly changing fields as genetics, hematology and immunology. The special language of electrocardiology, encephalography, neurology and psychology may baffle even the well-informed reader. Wide variation in the use of medical terms obviously hinders the communication of new findings and ideas. To bring order out of the linguistic chaos, a group of experts on medical terminology and medical dictionaries recently proposed that an international clearinghouse be established. This center would seek to standardize the language used by doctors the world over.

CONFUSION OF MEDICAL TERMS. The recommendation is presented in *Medical Terminology and Lexicography,* a volume published in Basel, Switzerland. The book contains the proceedings of a meeting convened in November 1965 by the Council for International Organizations of Medical Sciences (CIOMS), which was formed eighteen years ago under the auspices of UNESCO and the World Health Organization.

Citing many instances of the prevailing confusion in terminology, the CIOMS group emphasizes the difficulties created by a host of synonyms and eponyms differing from country to country. For example, *Candida albicans* has been discussed in medical writings under more than 170 names.

The chief languages of medicine today are English, French, German, Russian and Spanish. The CIOMS group offers the following estimate of the potential scientific readership in various languages: English, 2,650,000; German, 1,643,000; Russian, 1,231,000; French, 1,206,000; Chinese, 463,000; and Spanish, 361,000. The report indicated that 3,597 journals are published, and they carry a total of 221,000 articles each year.

Editors, translators and publishers of medical literature, particularly medical journals, play an important role in medical terminology. This has not been sufficiently appreciated.

STRICTER EDITING ADVISED. "Many medical publishers do not discharge their responsibilities to the medical profession satisfactorily," the language experts maintain. "Many medical journals still do not employ professional editors to edit articles before publication and leave it entirely to the authors to choose their terminology, even though their choice may violate existing international recommendations."

The development of a standardized terminology is a consummation devoutly to be wished and apparently hopeless to achieve. The terminology committee of the College of Sciences in Paris recommended that the word "malnutrition" be abolished, but it would be just as difficult to abolish the word as the condition it describes.

The time is far distant when a consensus is likely to be reached by qualified experts in lexicography, let alone by millions of medical practitioners in many countries. The situation continues to be a confused one, particularly when the language used by most scientists, namely English, seems to be least adequately represented in developing the proposed guides. In the publications of the leading American presses a translation of foreign quotations usually is included. When an author wishes to use a foreign quotation, it is well for him to insert a translation in parentheses.

Another frequent abuse of foreign terminology is the mixture of Latin and English terms in the writing of prescriptions, in anatomic descriptions and in the presentation of anatomic diagnoses associated with the records of postmortem examinations. Most American presses do not insist that authors use English names for diseases or for parts of the body. When an English term is available, however, its use is urged. When a Latin anatomic name is used, the Basle Nomina Anatomica (BNA) term should be employed if one is available.

Gender of Pronouns

In a novel or a literary essay, it may be natural to personify animals and to speak of them as "he" and "she." In scientific writing, however, in which an author is describing animals used in experiments in the laboratory, personification is not desirable, and the pronouns "it" and "which" should be used. The possessive form of the relative pronoun, "whose," may be used instead of "of which" or "in which" in references either to animals or to inanimate objects when awkwardness might result from insertion of a prepositional phrase.

Eponyms

In an article on gastrectomy, Sir Heneage Ogilvie[8] demonstrated the folly of depending on eponyms to designate a type of surgical procedure.

> There is no standard gastrectomy; but a gastrectomy for ulcer must satisfy three requirements: (1) it must reduce the production of

---

[8]Ogilvie, Sir Heneage: Gastrectomy: A human experiment, *Lancet, 253*:377, Sept. 13, 1947.

acid to a safe level and restrict its flow to the time when food is in the stomach; (2) it must ensure a certain period of gastric digestion and not throw the food straight from the oesophagus into the small intestine; and (3) it must direct the outflow from the stomach in an onward direction only. These requirements are satisfied by the Schoemaker type of Billroth I gastrectomy with end-to-end gastroduodenal anastomosis, and (if we must have names, let credit be properly attributed) by the high posterior Finsterer-Lake-Lahey modification of the Miculicz-Kronlein-Hofmeister-Reichel-Polya improvement of the Billroth II gastrectomy with a large valve and a small stoma.

The following terms to indicate tests or reactions appeared on one page of an article on tables: Cheyne-Stokes, Babinski, Strümpell, Marie-Foix and Klippel-Weil. While it is historically interesting to have a sign, test, reaction or disease known by the name of its discoverer, it is in the interest of scientific medicine to use a descriptive term. Certainly "reflex rigidity of the pupil" is better than "the Argyll Robertson pupil"; "great toe reflex" is preferable to "the Babinski sign"; "exophthalmic goiter" is more descriptive than "Basedow's disease." When a discovery is credited to several writers, the matter becomes complicated by the fact that national pride may assign a different name to the disease in several different countries. What is known in England as "Graves's disease" is called "Basedow's disease" on the Continent, except in Italy, where it is known as "Flajani's disease."

In some instances, nevertheless, a condition of disease may be recognized as an entity before its nature is sufficiently well defined to permit choice of an accurately descriptive name. "Hodgkin's disease," for instance, is at present preferable to "lymphogranuloma," "lymphogranulomatosis," "infectious granuloma" and other synonyms that have been proposed.

The following table of eponymic diseases is quoted from the *Standard Nomenclature of Diseases and Operations*[9]:

Abrami's disease. *See* Hemolytic icterus, acquired, 252 (9)
Acosta's disease. *See* Hypobaropathy, 113 (4)
Adams-Stokes syndrome: *Manifestation*, 246. *Diagnose disease,* e.g., Arteriosclerotic heart disease, 228 (5.0)

---

[9] The *Standard Nomenclature of Diseases and Operations* was published by The Blakiston Division, McGraw-Hill Book Company, Inc. for the American Medical Association. The latest edition appeared in 1961.

Addison's anemia. *See* Anemia, pernicious, 249 (7)
Addison's disease. *See* Tuberculosis of adrenal gland with cortical hypofunction, 454 (1); Adrenal cortical hypofunction, adrenal disease undetermined, 455 (7)
Adie syndrome. *See* Encephalomyelopathy of unknown origin, 464 (y); *manifestation,* 521
Albers-Schönberg disease. *See* Osteopetrosis (marble bones), 144 (0)
Albright's disease. *See* Osteitis fibrosa cystica, 150 (7)
Alzheimer's disease. *See* Presenile sclerosis, 101 (7); 480 (7)
Aran-Duchenne muscular atrophy. *See* Duchenne-Aran muscular atrophy
Argyll Robertson pupil. *See* Paralysis of intrinsic muscles of eye, 517; *and* Reflex rigidity of pupil, 519
Arnold-Chiari syndrome. *See* Caudal displacement of brain stem, cerebellum and spinal cord, 461 (0)
Arthus' phenomenon. *See* Anaphylactic reaction, generalized, 110 (3); *and* Anaphylactic reaction, local, 118 (3)
Avellis paralysis. *See* Paralysis, ambiguospinothalamic, 518; 521
Ayerza's syndrome. *See* Syphilis of pulmonary artery, 237 (1); Dilatation of pulmonary artery due to mitral stenosis, 238 (6); Hypertension of lesser circulation due to disease of lungs, 237 (4); Arteriosclerosis of lesser circulation, 238 (9)

Babinski-Nageotte syndrome, 522
Baker's cyst. *Diagnose* Popliteal bursitis under *Bursitis* due to unknown cause, 165 (9)
Bamberger-Marie disease. *See* Marie-Bamberger disease
Banti's disease. *See* Splenomegaly of undetermined origin, 256 (y)
Barcoo disease. *See* Veldt sore, 136 (9)
Barlow's disease. *See* Scurvy, 115 (7)
Barré-Guillain syndrome. *See* Guillain-Barré syndrome, 522
Basedow's disease. *See* Toxic diffuse goiter, 445 (9)
Baumgarten-Cruveilhier cirrhosis. *See* Cruveilhier-Baumgarten cirrhosis
Bazin's disease. *See* Tuberculosis indurativa (erythema induratum), 127 (1)
Bechterew's disease. *See* Arthritis, rheumatoid, of spine, 155 (1)
Bell's palsy. *See* Neuropathy of facial nerve due to pressure, 504 (4); *or* Neuropathy due to undetermined cause, 506 (y)
Benedikt syndrome. *See* Paralysis, mesencephalic, tegmental, 518; 521
von Bergmann's hypopituitarism. *See* Juvenile hypopituitarism, 451 (7)
Bernard-Horner syndrome. *See* Horner syndrome
Bernhardt's disease. *See* Meralgia paresthetica, 504 (4)
Besnier-Boeck disease. *See* Sarcoidosis, generalized, 109 (1)
Best's disease. *See* Degeneration, macular, congenital, 550 (0)
von Bezold's abscess. *See* Subperiosteal abscess of temporal bone, 601

72   *Medical Writing*

Bielschowsky-Jansky disease. *See* Amaurotic familial idiocy, late infantile, 463 (7)
Biermer's disease. *See* Anemia, pernicious, 249 (7)
Boeck's sarcoid. *See* Sarcoidosis, generalized, 109 (1) ; Sarcoidosis of region, 117 (1) ; Sarcoidosis cutis, 127 (1)
Bornholm disease. *See* Pleurodynia, epidemic, 205 (1)
Bouillaud's syndrome. *See* Rheumatic fever, 109 (1)
Bouveret's syndrome. *See* Auricular paroxysmal tachycardia due to unknown cause, 224 (x)
Bowen's disease, 134 (8)
   of lymph node, secondary, 260 (8)
   of mouth, 264 (8)
   of nasal mucosa, 178 (8)
Breda's disease. *See* Yaws, 110 (1) ; 126 (1)
Bright's disease. *See* under Nephritis
Brill's disease. *See* Typhus, 110 (1)
Brown-Séquard syndrome, 521
Buerger's disease. *See* Thromboangiitis obliterans, 233 (9)
Buschke's scleredema. *See* Scleredema adultorum, 136 (9)

Calvé-Perthes disease. *See* Legg-Calvé-Perthes disease
Carrion's disease. *See* Oroya fever, 109 (1) or Verruga peruana, 127 (1)
Cestan syndrome, 522
Cestan-Chenais paralysis. *See* Paralysis, medullary, tegmental, 518
Chagas' disease. *See* Trypanosomiasis, American, 110 (1)
Charcot joint. *See* Neurogenic arthropathy, 161 (5.5)
Charcot's syndrome. *Diagnose* Angiospasm of arteries of leg and foot, 232 (5.0)
Charcot-Marie-Tooth disease. *See* Progressive neuropathic (peroneal) muscular atrophy, 497 (9)
Cheadle's disease. *See* Scurvy, 115 (7)
Chenais-Cestan paralysis. *See* Cestan-Chenais paralysis
Chiari-Arnold syndrome. *See* Caudal displacement of brain stem, cerebellum and spinal cord, 461 (0)
Christian-Schüller disease, 114 (7)
Christian-Weber disease. *See* Nodular, nonsuppurative panniculitis, 126 (1)
Clark's paralysis. See Paralysis, cerebral, infantile, 518
Clarke-Hadfield syndrome. *See* Pancreatic infantilism, 327 (0)
Claude syndrome, 522
Coats's disease. *See* Retinitis exudative, 553, (5.0)
Colles' fracture, 148 (4)
Cooley's anemia. *See* Familial erythroblastic anemia, 250 (9)
Costen's syndrome complex. *See* Impaired hearing due to malocclusion of

temporomandibular joint; *and* Otalgia due to malocclusion of temporomandibular joint, 589 (6)

Crohn's disease. *See* Ileitis, regional, 304 (9)

Crouzon's disease. *See* Hypertelorism, 143 (0)

Cruveilhier's disease. *See* Progressive myelopathic muscular atrophy, 497 (9)

Cruveilhier- Baumgarten cirrhosis. *See* Cirrhosis of liver, congenital, 318 (0)

Curling's ulcer. *See* Duodenal ulcer due to burns, 301 (4)

Cushing's disease. *See* Changes in bone associated with pituitary basophilism, 150 (7); Pituitary basophilism, 451 (7); Adrenal cortical hyperfunction, 455 (7)

Dana-Putnam syndrome. *See* Putnam-Dana syndrome

Darier's disease. *See* Keratosis follicularis, 124 (0)

Darier-Roussy sarcoid, 136 (9)

Darling's histoplasmosis. *See* Histoplasmosis, 110 (2)

Déjerine-Landouzy atrophy. *See* Landouzy-Déjerine atrophy

Déjerine-Roussy syndrome, 522

Déjerine-Sottas neuropathy. *See* Progressive hypertrophic interstitial neuropathy, 509 (9)

Dercum's disease. *See* Adiposis dolorosa, 114 (7)

Devic's disease. *See* Optic neuroencephalomyelopathy, 464 (9)

Dietl's crisis. *See* Angulation of ureter, 349 (6)

Dieulafoy's ulcer. *See* Erosion of stomach, 292 (9)

Dresbach's syndrome. *See* Sickle cell anemia, 252 (9)

Duchenne-Aran muscular atrophy. *See* Myelopathic muscular atrophy, 497 (9)

Duhring's disease. *See* Dermatitis herpetiformis, 135 (9)

Dupuytren's contracture, 174 (9)

Durand-Nicolas-Favre disease. *See* Lymphogranuloma, veneral, 259 (1)

Economo's disease. *See* Encephalitis, epidemic, acute, lethargic type, 476 (1)

Engman's disease. *See* Dermatitis infectiosa eczematoides, 125 (1)

Erb's dystrophy. *See* Pseudohypertrophic muscular dystrophy, 169 (9)

Erb's palsy. *See under* Birth injury: laceration of peripheral nerve, 501 (0)

Erb's paralysis. *See* Paralysis, syphilitic, spastic, spinal, 492 (1); Pseudohypertrophic muscular dystrophy, 169 (9)

Erb-Goldflam disease. *See* Myasthenia gravis, 168 (5.5)

Eulenburg's disease. *See* Paramyotonia congenita, 166 (0)

Ewing's tumor. *See* Angioendothelioma, 150 (8)

Faber's syndrome. *See* Anemia, hypochromic, 249 (7)

Fahr-Volhard's disease. *See* Arteriolar nephrosclerosis, advanced stage; malignant nephrosclerosis, 344 (5.0)

Fallot, tetralogy of. *See* Ventricular septal defect, pulmonary stenosis or atresia, dextraposition of aorta and hypertrophy of right ventricle, 211 (0)
Fanconi's disease. *See* Constitutional infantile anemia resembling pernicious anemia, 248 (0)
Favre-Durand-Nicolas disease. *See* Lymphogranuloma, venereal, 259 (1)
Feer's disease. *See* Erythredema polyneuropathy, 505 (x)
Feil-Klippel syndrome, *Diagnose* Deformity of bone, 144 (1) ; Tuberculosis of spine, 146 (1)
Felty's syndrome. *See* Rheumatoid arthritis, 155 (1)
Fiedler's myocarditis. *See* Acute isolated myocarditis due to unknown cause, 223 (9)
Flajani's disease. *See* Toxic diffuse goiter, 445 (9)
Flatau-Schilder disease. *See* Schilder's disease
Fleischer-Kayser ring. *See* Kayser-Fleischer ring
Fordyce's disease of mouth. *See* Sebaceous glands of mucocutaneous junction aberrant, 124 (0)
Fordyce-Fox disease, 135 (9)
Foville syndrome, 522
Fox-Fordyce disease, 135 (9)
Francis disease. *See* Tularemia, 110 (1)
Frank's capillary toxicosis. *See* Nonthrombopenic purpura, cause unknown, 243 (x)
Frei's disease. *See* Lymphogranuloma, venereal, 259 (1)
Freiberg's infraction of metatarsal head. *See* Osteochondrosis of head of metatarsal bone, 152 (9)
Friderichsen-Waterhouse syndrome. *See* Waterhouse-Friderichsen syndrome
Friedreich's ataxia. *See* Hereditary sclerosis, spinal form, 483 (9)
Froehlich's syndrome. *See* Sex infantilism with obesity (adiposogenital dystrophy), 451 (7)
Fuchs' black spot. *See* Choroidal changes in myopia, 541 (4)
Fuchs' conus. *See* Conus, oblique, 556 (0)

Garre's disease. *See* Osteitis, sclerotic nonsuppurative, 145 (1)
Gaucher's disease, 114 (7)
Gee's disease. *See* Celiac disease, 262 (x)
Gelineau's syndrome. *See* Narcolepsy, 485 (x)
Ghon tubercle. *See* Tuberculosis of lung, childhood type, 199 (1)
von Gierke's disease. *See* Glycogenosis, 114 (7) ; 223 (7)
Gilford-Hutchinson disease. *See* Hutchinson-Gilford disease
Glisson's disease. *See* Rickets, 115 (7)
Goldflam-Erb disease. *See* Myasthenia gravis, 168 (5.5)
Gowers' syndrome. *See* Paroxysmal vasovagal attacks, 484 (x)
Gradenigo syndrome, 522. *See* also Extradural abscess involving petrous bone, 600

Grave's disease. *See* Toxic diffuse goiter, 445 (9)
Gubler-Millard paralysis. *See* Millard-Gubler paralysis
Guillain-Barré syndrome, 522
Gull's disease. *See* Atrophy of thyroid gland with myxedema, 445 (9)
Gull and Sutton's disease. *See* Arteriosclerosis, generalized, 233 (9)

Hadfield-Clarke syndrome. *See* Clarke-Hadfield syndrome
Haff disease. *See* Poisoning, general, with arsenic, 111 (3)
Hallopeau's acrodermatitis. *See* Acrodermatitis continua, 125 (1)
Hanot's disease. *See* Hypertrophic cirrhosis, 321 (9)
Hansen's disease. *See* Leprosy, 109 (1)
Haverhill fever, 109 (1)
Heberden's nodes. *See* Degenerative joint disease, multiple, due to unknown cause, 162 (9)
Hebra's disease. *See* Erythema multiforme exudativum, 135 (9)
Hebra's pityriasis. *See* Pityriasis rubra, 136 (9)
Henle's warts. *See* Hyalin formation in cornea (by endothelial cells), 533 (7)
Henoch's purpura. *See* Nonthrombopenic purpura, cause unknown, 243 (x)
Herrick's anemia. *See* Sickle cell anemia, 252 (9)
Hirschsprung's disease. *See* Dilatation of colon, congenital, megacolon, congenital, 305 (0)
Hodgkin's disease, 261 (9)
Hodgkin's disease of skin, 135 (9)
Hoffmann-Werdnig syndrome. *See* Hereditary familial spinal muscular atrophy, 497 (9)
Horner's syndrome, 522. *See* also Cervical sympathetic paralysis, 507 (4); Enophthalmos due to paralysis of sympathetic innervation, 528 (5.5)
Horton's syndrome. *See* Histamine headache, 472 (5.5)
Hunner's ulcer. *See* Interstitial cystitis with ulceration, 356 (9)
Huntington's chorea. *See* Hereditary chronic progressive chorea, 483 (9)
Hurler's disease. *See* Lipochondrodystrophy, 108 (0)
Hutchinson-Boeck disease. *See* Sarcoidosis, generalized, 109 (1)
Hutchinson-Gilford disease. *See* Progeria, 115 (7)
Hyde's disease. *See* Prurigo nodularis, 136 (9)

Jacksonian epilepsy. *See* Focal, motor or sensory, cortical seizures, 484 (x)
Jackson's veil or membrane. *See* Peritoneal adhesions and bands, congenital, 330 (0)
von Jaksch's' anemia. *A more specific diagnosis is to be made*
Janet's disease. *See* Psychasthenia, 104
Jansky-Bielschowsky disease. *See* Bielschowsky-Jansky disease
Jensen's disease. *See* Retinochoroiditis juxtapapillaris, 551 (1)

Kahler's disease. *See* Myeloma, 250 (8)
Kaposi's disease. *See* Xeroderma pigmentosum, 124 (0)

Kaposi's sarcoma. *See* Multiple idiopathic hemorrahagic sarcoma, 134 (8)
Kayser-Fleischer ring. *See* Pigment deposit in limbus, 534 (9)
Kienböck's disease. *See* Osteochondrosis of lunate bone, 152 (9)
Klippel-Feil syndrome. *Diagnose* Deformity of bone, 144 (1); Tuberculosis of spine, 146 (1)
Koch-Weeks bacillus. *See* Hemophilus influenzae, 62
Koch-Weeks conjunctivitis. *See* Influenzal conjunctivitis, 584 (1)
Köhler's bone disease. *See* Osteochondrosis of navicular, 152 (9)
Korsakoff's psychosis, 100 (3)
Krabbe's disease. *See* Diffuse, infantile familial cerebral sclerosis, 483 (9)
Kraepelin-Morel disease. *See* Morel-Kraepelin disease
Krukenberg's spindle. *See* Melanosis of cornea, following uveitis, 530 (1); Melanosis of cornea, due to myopia, 532 (4)
Krukenberg's tumor. *See* Fibrosarcoma mucocellulare carcinomatodes, 414 (8)
Kümmell's disease. *See* Compression fracture of vertebra, *under* Fracture, compression, 147 (4)
Kussmaul's disease. *See* Periarteritis nodosa, 231 (1)

Laennec's cirrhosis, 321 (9)
Landouzy-Déjerine atrophy. *See* Facioscapulohumeral atrophy, 169 (9)
Landry's paralysis. *See* Myelitis, ascending, acute, 491 (1)
de Lange's syndrome. *See* Dystrophia myotonica, 170 (9)
Launois' syndrome. *See* Hypophysial gigantism, 451 (7)
Laurence-Moon-Biedl syndrome, 108 (0)
Leber's optic atrophy. *See* Hereditary optic atrophy, 505 (9); 559 (9)
Legg-Calvé-Perthes disease. *See* Osteochondrosis of capital epiphysis of femur, 152 (9)
Lewandowsky's disease. *See* Tuberculid (rosacea-like), 127 (1)
Leyden-Moebius' dystrophy. *See* Progressive muscular dystrophy, 169 (9)
Lichtheim's syndrome. *See* Dorsolateral spinal degeneration, 496 (7)
Little's disease. *See* Cerebral spastic infantile paralysis, 475 (0)
Lobstein's disease. *See* Fragilitas ossium, 143 (0)
Lorain syndrome. *See* Dwarfism and infantilism, 451 (7)
Ludwig's anginia. *See* Cellulitis of floor of mouth, 263 (1)

Madelung's deformity. *See* Radius, idiopathic progressive curvature of, 142 (0)
Majocchi's disease. *See* Purpura annularis telangiectodes, 132 (5.0)
Marfan's syndrome. *See* Arachnodactyly, 108 (0)
Marie's sclerosis. *See* Hereditary sclerosis, cerebellar form, 483 (9)
Marie's syndrome. *See* Acromegaly, 451 (7)
Marie-Bamberger disease. *See* Secondary hypertrophic osteoarthropathy, 149 (7)

Marie-Strümpell arthritis. *See* Arthritis, rheumatoid, of spine, 155 (1)
Marie-Tooth disease. *See* Charcot-Marie-Tooth disease.
Ménière's syndrome, 599 (x) ; 522
Merzbacher-Pelizaeus disease. *See* Aplasia axialis extracorticalis congenita, 474 (0)
Mikulicz's disease. *See* Hypertrophy of salivary glands, 277 (9) ; Achroacytosis of lacrimal gland, due to infection, 580 (1) tuberculous, 580 (1) ; due to unknown cause, 583 (9)
Millard-Gubler paralysis. *See* Paralysis, alternating, abducens, facial, hemiplegic, 517
Milroy's edema. *See* Familial hereditary edema, 137 (x)
Mitchell's disease. *See* Erythromelalgia, 232 (5.5)
Moebius-Leyden's dystrophy. *See* Leyden-Moebius' dystrophy
Mönckberg's arteriosclerosis. *See* Arteriosclerosis, medial, especially with calcification, 233 (9)
Moon-Laurence-Biedl syndrome, 108 (0)
Mooren's ulcer. *See* Ulcer, rodent, of cornea, 530 (1)
Morax-Axenfeld conjunctivitis. *See* Conjunctivitis due to Hemophilus duplex (Morax-Axenfeld bacillus), 584 (1)
Morel-Kraepelin disease. *See* Dementia precox, 102 (x)
Morgagni's hydatid. *See* Cyst of oviduct, congenital, 408 (0)
Morquio's disease. *See* Eccentro-osteochondrodysplasia, 143 (0)
Morvan's disease. *See* Syringomyelia, 496 (8)

Nägele's pelvis, 434 (4)
Nageotte-Babinski syndrome. *See* Babinski-Nageotte syndrome, 522
Nicolas-Favre-Durand disease. *See* Lymphogranuloma, venereal, 259 (1)
Niemann-Pick disease, 114 (7)

Oguchi's disease. *See* Night blindness, congenital (Japanese), 551 (0)
Ollier's disease. *See* Dyschondroplasia, 143 (0)
Oppenheim's disease. *See* Amyotonia congenita, 490 (0)
Oppenheim-Urbach disease. *See* Urbach-Oppenheim disease
Osgood-Schlatter disease. *See* Osteochondrosis of tuberosity of tibia, 152 (9)
Osler-Vaquez disease. *See* Polycythemia, primary; erythremia, 250 (7)

Paget's disease of bone. *See* Osteitis deformans, 151 (9)
Paget's disease of nipple. *See* Carcinoma simplex of nipple, 140 (8)
Parinaud's conjunctivitis. *See* Leptotrichosis of conjunctiva, 585 (2)
Parinaud syndrome, 522
Parkinson's disease. *See* Paralysis agitans, 483 (9)
Parry's disease. *See* Toxic diffuse goiter, 445 (9)
Pelizaeus-Merzbacher disease. *See* Merzbacher-Pelizaeus disease
Pellegrini-Stieda disease. *See* Calcification of medial collateral ligament of knee due to trauma, 156 (4)

Perthes' disease. *See* Legg-Calvé-Perthes disease
Peyronie's disease. *See* Induration of corpora cavernosa, 3689 (9)
Pfeiffer's disease. *See* Mononucleosis, infectious, 109 (1)
Pick's (Friedel Pick) disease. *See* Polyserositis, 335 (9)
Pick-Niemann disease, 114 (7)
Plummer-Vinson syndrome. *See* Anemia, hypochromic, 249 (7); Anemia secondary to iron starvation, 252 (7)
Poncet's disease. *Diagnose* Arthritis due to infection, multiple tuberculous, 154 (1)
Pott's disease. *See* Tuberculosis of vertebra, 146 (1)
Pott's fracture, 148 (4). *The criterion is disruption of the inferior tibiofibular joint. It is better to classify this fracture in accordance with the specific lesions present:* e.g., Fracture of tibia, internal malleolus, 147 (4); Fracture of shaft of fibula, lower third, 147 (4); Tear of inferior tibiofibular ligament, 158 (4)
Putnam-Dana syndrome. *See* Dorsolateral sclerosis; manifestation, 522. *Diagnose disease*

Queyrat's erythroplasia, buccal, 134, (8); 264 (8); lingual, 134 (8); 268 (8); vulvar, 134 (8); 392 (8); of glans penis, 367 (8); of prepuce, 367 (8)
Quincke's disease. *See* Angioneurotic edema, 132 (5.5); 242 (5.5)

Raynaud's disease, 232 (5.5)
von Recklinghausen's disease. *See* Neurofibromatosis, 135 (8)
von Recklinghausen's disease of bone. *See* Osteitis fibrosa cystica, generalized, 150 (7)
Riedel's lobe. *See* Lobulation of liver, abnormal, congenital, 318 (0)
Riedel's struma. *See* Thyroiditis, chronic, 445 (9)
Ritter's disease. *See* Dermatitis exfoliativa, 135 (9)
Robert's pelvis, 435 (9)
Roger's disease. *See* Ventricular septal defect, localized, 212 (0)
Rokitansky's disease. *See* Acute yellow atrophy of liver, 321 (9)
Roussy-Darier sarcoid, 136 (9)
Roussy-Déjerine syndrome. *See* Déjerine-Roussy syndrome, 522

St. Vitus dance. *See* Chorea, 476 (1)
Schamberg's disease. *See* Dermatosis, progressive, pigmentary, 131 (5.0)
Schaumann's syndrome. *See* Sarcoidosis, generalized, 109 (1)
Schilder's disease. *See* Progressive subcortical encephalopathy, 483 (9)
Schimmelbusch's disease. *See* Cystic breast due to unknown cause, 139 (6)
Schlatter-Osgood disease. *See* Osteochondrosis of tuberosity of tibia, 152 (9)
Schmorl's disease. *See* Herniation of nucleus pulposus, cause unknown, 162 (9)
Schönlein's disease. *See* Nonthrombopenic purpura, cause unknown, 243 (x)

Schüller-Christian disease, 114 (7)
Senear-Usher disease. See Pemphigus erythematosus, 136 (9)
Siemens' syndrome. See Defect, congenital ectodermal, 123 (0)
Simmonds' disease. See Hypopituitary cachexia, 451 (7)
Sottas-Déjerine neuropathy. See Déjerine-Sottas neuropathy
Spielmeyer-Stock disease. See Atrophy, retinal, in juvenile amaurotic familial idiocy, 555 (9)
Spielmeyer-Vogt disease. See Amaurotic familial idiocy, juvenile 463 (7)
Sprengel's deformity. See Scapula, congenital elevation of, 143 (0)
Stahl's pigment line. See Linea corneae senilis, 533 (7)
Stieda-Pellegrini disease. See Pellegrini-Stieda disease
Still's disease. See Arthritis, rheumatoid, multiple, 155 (1)
Stock-Spielmeyer disease. See Spielmeyer-Stock disease
Stokes-Adams syndrome: *manifestation,* 246. *Diagnose disease,* e.g., Arteriosclerotic heart disease, 228 (5.0)
Strümpell-Marie disease. *Diagnose* Rheumatoid arthritis of Spine, under Arthritis, rheumatoid, 155 (1)
Strümpell-Westphal pseudosclerosis. See Pseudosclerosis, 483 (9)
Sudeck's atrophy. See Osteoporosis due to trauma, 148 (4)
Sutton and Gull's disease. See Gull and Sutton's disease
Sydenham's chorea. See Chorea, 476 (1)

Tay's choroiditis. See Drusen of choroid, 542 (9)
Tay-Sach's disease. See Amaurotic familial idiocy, infantile, 463 (7); Atrophy, retinal, in infantile amaurotic familial idiocy, 555 (9)
Tetralogy of Fallot. See Ventricular septal defect, pulmonary stenosis or atresia, dextraposition of aorta and hypertrophy of right ventricle, 211 (0)
Thomsen's disease. See Myotonia congenita, 166 (0)

Urbach-Oppenheim disease. See Necrobiosis lipoidica diabeticorum, 133 (7)
Usher-Senear disease. See Senear-Usher disease

Vaquez-Osler disease. See Polycythemia, primary; erythremia, 250 (7)
Vernet syndrome, 522
Villaret syndrome, 522
Vincent's angina, 127 (1)
Vincent's infection of larynx, 185 (1); of bronchus, 193 (1); of mouth, 263 (1); of tongue, 267 (1); of tonsil, 281 (1); of lingual tonsil, 282 (1)
Vinson-Plummer syndrome. See Plummer-Vinson syndrome
Vogt-Spielmeyer disease. See Spielmeyer-Vogt disease
Volhard-Fahr's disease. See Fahr-Volhards' disease
Volkmann's contracture. See Contracture due to ischemia, 168 (5.0)
Vossius' ring, 545 (4)

Waterhouse-Friderichsen syndrome. *See* Meningitis, cerebrospinal, epidemic (meningococcic), 468 (1)
Weber's paralysis. *See* Paralysis, alternating, oculomotor, hemiplegic, 518
Weber-Christian disease. *See* Nodular, nonsuppurative panniculitis, 126 (1)
Weil's disease. *See* Jaundice, spirochetal, 109 (1)
Werdnig-Hoffmann syndrome. *See* Hoffmann-Werdnig syndrome
Werlhof's disease. *See* Thrombopenic purpura; idiopathic hemorrhagic purpura, 252 (7)
Wernicke's disease. *See* Polioencephalitis, superior, hemorrhagic, 477 (1)
Westphal-Strümpell pseudosclerosis. *See* Strümpell-Westphal pseudosclerosis
Whitmore's disease. *See* Melioidosis, 110 (1)
Wilms' tumor. *See* Embryonal carcinosarcoma of kidney, 345 (8)
Wilson's hepatolenticular degeneration. *See* Hepatolenticular degeneration, 483 (9)

Antepartum and Prenatal

In the periodicals published by the American Medical Association a distinction is made between these two words. "Antepartum" is used to refer to the mother before parturition or to events or circumstances affecting her during pregnancy; "prenatal," to refer to the fetus before birth.

Epidemic Encephalitis

In order to avoid the confusion occasioned by using "epidemic encephalitis" to refer to all types of acute encephalitis, it is well to employ "lethargic encephalitis" or "encephalitis lethargica" to designate the disease originally described by von Economo in order to distinguish it from the types observed in epidemics in St. Louis, Toledo (Ohio) and Japan.

Nomenclature of Fungous Diseases

Mycology is one of the newer branches of medicine, and the confusion and inconsistency evident in some of the terms relating to fungous diseases are only now being corrected. An author should be guided by the nomenclature adopted by scientific bodies concerned with medical mycology and should observe the usages of present authorities in that field. The following definitions represent the trend of current usage. "Dermatomycosis" is a generic term including all infections due to fungi, superficial and deep. "Dermatophytosis" is synonymous with "dermatomycosis," but usage tends to associate "dermatophytosis" with ringworm of the hands and feet or with superficial fungous infections of the skin. "Epidermophytosis," "trichophytosis" and similar words indicate infection due to *Epidermophyton, Trichophyton* or some other specific fungus. "Dermatophytid" refers to a lesion of an allergic reaction to a dermatophytosis.

Lymphogranuloma Venereum

The American Medical Association, as well as the National Conference on Nomenclature of Disease, prefers the term "lymphogranuloma venereum" to "inguinal lymphogranuloma," "lymphogranuloma inguinale" or "lymphopathia venerea (um)."

This disease and its name should not be confused with inguinal granuloma (granuloma inguinale).

-Derma

Names of cutaneous diseases properly end in "-derma" (neuter gender), as "scleroderma circumscriptum." The use of "-dermia" is unwarranted.

Mongolians, Mongoloids

Some authors have objected to the term "mongolian idiot" because, they say, some of the persons affected have intelligence above the level of idiocy. For this reason they have wished to use "mongolian" or "mongoloid" as a noun to replace "mongolian idiot." In addition to the undesirability of the use of an adjective as a noun, neither designation is accurate, for "mongolian" in its strict sense applies to a member of the Mongol or of a similar race and "mongoloid" connotes particularly the physical characteristics. The difficulties seem to be avoided if one uses "mongolism" as the name for the condition and speaks of the persons affected as "persons with mongolism." (Though "mongolism" is preferable to "mongolian idiocy," the latter, as well as "mongolian idiot," may be used if an author wishes.) The eponymic designation is Down's disease.

Infection vs. Infestation

In accordance with the report of a specially assigned committee of the American Society of Parasitologists, the word "infection" is used with regard to bacteria, protozoa and helminths, while the word "infestation" is reserved for invasion by arthropods, including ticks, mites and insects.

-Emia Words

Usage among physicians and the definitions in medical and in general dictionaries show great inconsistency in the significance attached to words ending in "-emia" and prefixed by "hyper-" or "hypo-." Sometimes an "-emia" is considered as the presence of a substance in the blood; sometimes, as an excess; sometimes, even as an abnormally small amount. Some authors always employ the prefix "hyper-" when they wish to state that an excess was present; others use the "-emia" word—for instance "glycemia"—alone. To avoid confusion it is well to use such words in the following manner:

Word	To Denote
"-emia" (e.g., lipemia)	presence of a substance in the blood
"hyper—emia" (e.g., hyperglycemia)	presence of an excess
"hypo—emia" (e.g., hypocholesteremia)	presence of an abnormally small amount

Official Nomenclature

Certain scientific bodies, including the American Chemical Society, the International Zoological Congress, the Bureau of the Census, the American Roentgenologic Association, the National Conference on Nomenclature of Disease and the German Anatomical Society in Basle, Switzerland, which published the Basle Nomina Anatomica, have adopted official codes of nomenclature. Ordinarily it is advisable to employ the terms and spellings established by such organizations. The *Standard Nomenclature of Diseases and Operations* is a periodically revised authority in its field.

6
SPELLING

SPELLING should be consistent; the writer should follow a definite style, preferably that adopted by the periodical to which he wishes to submit a manuscript. Some publications follow conservative spelling; others have adopted reformed spelling. Many medical publishers make it a practice to follow *Blakiston's New Gould Medical Dictionary* or Dorland's *The American Illustrated Medical Dictionary* as standards for medical terms and *Webster's New International Dictionary* or *Funk & Wagnalls New Standard Dictionary* for other words.

I prefer certain special usages, as listed here:[1]

abstracter	analogous	blennorrhea
accommodate	ancylostoma	bougienage
acinous	aneurysm	bromide
adaptable	angiitis	bromine
adenosine	ankylosis	burr
adiadokokinesis	appendectomy	calix
admissible	appendical	calorie
afterward	argentophilic (adj.)	calvaria
aline	arrhythmia	cannula
alinement	arsphenamine	cantaloup
alkalis	artefact	carotene
alkalization	ascendant (noun)	catabolism
alkalize	bacteremia	centrifugation
allotted	basophilic (adj.)	centrifuge (verb)
amebicide	benefited	chlorophyll
ampul	beside (by the side of)	cholangitis
anaerobic	besides (in addition to)	cholesteremia

---

[1] A few words concerning the spelling of which there is no inconsistency have been included in the list because they are frequently spelled incorrectly in manuscripts.

cholesterol
cholesterosis
choroid
cigaret
clue
cocaine
-coccic (adj. ending)
coccidioidal
combated
confrère
cooperation
criticize
critique
crystalline
curet
curettage
curettement
cyclothymic
débride
defense
demyelinate
demyelination
descendant (noun)
desiccate
devise* (verb)
diadokokinesis
dietitian
dilatation (state of being dilated)
dilation (act of dilating)
diphtheritic
discernible
disk
dispatch
distention
drachm
dulness
embarrass
embed
embryos
employee
enclosed

endameba
endochondral
endorse
eosinophilic (adj.)
epithelization
epithelize
exophthalmos
faker
fantasy
fantom†
fiber
fulfil
fulness
fungous (adj.)
fungus (noun)
gage
glycosuria
gray
grip
guaiacol
hemianopsia
hemopoietic
hiccup
hilus
homogenization
homogenize
hyalin (noun)
hyaline (adj.)
hypophysial
impracticable
inoculate
insanitary
insure
intern
intrachondrial
intravenous
intussusception
ipsilateral
lacrimal
leukemia
leukocyte
lymphangitis
lyophile
lyse*

lysozyme
malpighian
mamilla
mamillary
mammary
marasmic
microgliocytes
migraine
mold
mosquitoes
mucopus
mucous (adj.)
mucus (noun)
multilocular
mycotic
myelinate
myelination
myocardial
negligible
occurring
omental
ophthalmology
oxidase
papilledema
pavaex
pedicel (*bot.*, stem)
pedicle (*anat.*, vertebral process; *med.*, stem of tumor)
penile
periangiitis
periarticular
pericholangitis
perilymphangitis
perineural (around the nerve)
perineurial (referring to perineurium)
perisinal
perivascular
peroxidase
phagocytose

phlorhizin
phosphorus
physicochemical (pertaining to physical chemistry or to physics and chemistry)
physiochemical (pertaining to physiologic chemistry)
pipet
piriform, piriformis
pneumo- (of air)
pneumono- (of the lung)
pontile
practice
precox
premycotic
preventive
previa
prodrome
promoter
pruritus
psychoanalysis
putrefy
pyretic
pyrimidine
pyrrole
quinacrine (atabrine)

radical (adj.)
radical (*chem.*, group of atoms; *philol.*, part of word)
radicle (*anat.*, root or rootlike structure)
rale
raphe
reenforce
résumé
rhythm
rime
role
rosette*
sagittal
Salpêtrière
sanatorium
scirrhous (adj.)
scirrhus (noun)
serviceable
[sic]
sinal
skeptical
skilful
sprue
stable
streptotrichal
sulfhydril
sulfobromophthalein

supersede
technic
thermostable
thromboangiitis
thrombopenia
thrombopenic
timbre* (of tone)
titer
tonsillitis
toward
translator
tubercular (nodular)
tuberculous (pertaining to tuberculosis)
tuberous
unpractical
vacuolate
vacuolation
venipuncture
ventrifixation
verruca peruviana
verrucous
villous (adj.)
vitamin
-ward (suffix)
whisky
wilful
xanthophyll

SIMPLIFIED SPELLINGS

The following simplified spellings, which have been approved by a committee of the editors of the publications of the American Chemical Society, are recommended: *e* for *ae*, as in anesthetic, hemoglobin; *f* for *ph* in sulfur and the sulfur compounds; *f* for *gh*, as in draft; *et* for *ette*, as in pipet; *ze* for *se*, as in analyze; *l* for

---

*Exception to rule.

†When "phantom" is used in the sense of a model, as in "phantom experiments," the "ph" spelling should be used.

ll in words like distil (when the accent is on the last syllable the *l* is doubled in participles, as *distilled;* also in *mono*syllables, as *still); l* for *ll*, as in fulness; *e* for *oe,* as in pharmacopeia; *or* for *our,* as in behavior; *er* for *re,* as in fiber; and *mold* not *mould, gage* not *gauge,* and *role* not *rôle.*

For words ending in *"og"* or *"ogue,"* the form listed as preferred in *Blakiston's New Gould Medical Dictionary* or in Webster's *New International Dictionary* is used. If the *"og"* and the *"ogue"* forms are given as in equally good usage, the *"og"* spelling is chosen.

NAMES OF PERSONS

Special attention should be given to the spelling of names of persons. The American Medical Directory may be consulted for the names of physicians in the United States. Directories and lists of physicians of foreign countries are available in medical libraries. *Who's Who* may prove valuable. Names of well-known investigators are found in medical dictionaries. When an article or a book is consulted and cited, the author's name should be copied correctly, with special attention being given to the insertion of accents in a foreign name.

In the following list are a few names that are frequently misspelled:

Bence Jones, Henry
Berkefeld
Darkshevich
de Fortuyn, Droogleever
Déjerine
del Río-Hortega, Pío
Greifswald
Kjeldahl
Korsakoff
Küstner (Prausnitz-Küstner reaction)
Little, E. G. Graham
MacCallum, W. G.
McCollum, E. V.
Metchnikoff
Neelsen (Ziehl-Neelsen stain)
Pavlov
Rinne
Šafář
Schick, Béla
Shwartzman, Gregory (Shwartzman phenomenon)
Tallqvist
Van Gieson
Wassermann

GEOGRAPHIC NAMES

For the spelling of foreign geographic names, any recognized modern atlas or the list of the United Nations may be followed. When two spellings are given, the anglicized form is preferred.

In the following list are a few geographic names which are encountered frequently in manuscripts:

Berne (Switzerland)
Brussels (Belgium)
Czechoslovak (adj.)
Czechoslovakia
Danzig
Frankfort on the Main (Germany)
Göteborg (Sweden)
Leipzig (Germany)
Liége (Belgium)
Munich (Germany)
Netherland (adj.)
Netherland East Indies
Netherlands
Prague (Czechoslovakia)
Rumania
San Jose (Calif.)
San José (Costa Rica, Uruguay)
Serbia
Yugoslavia
Zurich (Switzerland)

Other rules concerning geographic names will be found in Chapter 8.

DIVISION OF WORDS INTO SYLLABLES

The following four rules have been established by *Funk & Wagnalls New Standard Dictionary* for the division of words:

Rule I. A consonant or a digraph or trigraph between two vowels goes into the later syllable when the first vowel is long, half-long or obscure (except -er as in gen-er-al) ; as, fa-tal, sea-son, sepa-rate, pro-gram, seda-tive, omi-nous, mecha-nism, pecu-liar, pro-phetic, medi-cal, practi-cal, fa-ther, me-tallic, mo-nopo-ly, pre-sent (v.), de-throne, ca-pacity, pro-gress (v.), ca-pable, proce-dure.

Rule II. A consonant between two vowels goes into the earlier syllable when the first vowel is short and has any stress; as, prod-uct, rap-id, pres-ent (n.), vis-it, ton-ic, bus-y, crit-ic, flor-id, char-ity, sep-arate.

Rule III. Adjoining consonants usually separate into two syllables; as, at-tract, con-demn, pam-phlet, syl-lable, prac-tical, moun-tain, infan-try, connec-tion, produc-tive, detec-tive, suc-ces-sor, defen-dant, cor-respon-dent, as-sis-tant, mat-ting, com-pel-ling, fret-ted, En-gland. However, doubled consonants ending a primitive

88   *Medical Writing*

word are kept together before a purely English suffix; as, tell-ing, hiss-ing.

Rule IV. Purely English suffixes (-ed, -er, -est, -eth, -ing, -ish, -y) are always kept distinct (except when the terminal letter of the primitive word is repeated, as in compel-ling) ; as heat-ed, hat-ed, bak-er, speak-er, speak-est, wak-eth, search-eth, hast-ing, baptiz-ing, brak-ing, break-ing, freak-ish, head-y. But terminations like -al, -ant, -ent, -ive, -or are treated as merely anglicized endings (usually of Latin or Greek words taken into English entire, but with terminal change), not as separable English suffixes. Thus such confusion as music-al, practi-cal, conjunc-tive, disjunct-ive, abundant, defend-ant, which is found in some other works, is avoided. The treatment here given makes every one of these terminations begin with the consonant.

HYPHENATION

Hyphens are not necessary when the meaning of double or compound words is clear without them. Some dictionaries use more hyphens than seem to be necessary for clearness.

A hyphen is not used with a prefix unless mispronunciation or ambiguity might result without it.[2] A prefix preceding a proper noun, as in "non" or "post" is followed by a word beginning with noun, as in "non-American," requires a hyphen. When "non" or "post" is followed by a word beginning with "n" (or an "n" sound) or "t," respectively, a hyphen should be used, as in "non-nitrogenous," "non-pneumatic" and "post-traumatic." Other prefixes ending in a consonant usually are joined without a hyphen to a word beginning with the same consonant. Occasionally one of the consonants is dropped. For the spelling of such words, the medical dictionaries mentioned or *Webster's New International Dictionary* should be consulted. A prefix of more than one syllable ending in a vowel should be hyphenated before the same vowel, as in "semi-

---

[2]It was formerly the rule of the American Medical Association Press to hyphenate all prefixes of more than one syllable ending in "a" or "o" when followed by a vowel. Since the application of this principle led to inconsistency between the forms of similar words and between the spellings thus devised and those given in most of the standard dictionaries, this practice has been discontinued except when ambiguity or mispronunciation might result from omission of the hyphen.

isolated" and "hypo-ovarian," except in chemical or other pharmaceutic names. One should write "endoderm and ectoderm" rather than "endo- and ectoderm."

When two similar vowels come together in the name of a drug, the name is not hyphenated, as in paraaminobenzoic acid. The prefix "co" when used to refer to an agent is hyphenated; i.e., co-worker, co-author. When "co" refers to a state or condition, the word is written without a hyphen; i.e. coexistent.

A few general rules governing the formation of compounds of certain types may be given. (These rules do not apply, of course, to words, such as "background," which have long been established as one word and are so listed in general dictionaries.)

Compounds

1. Compounds in which the second member represents an agent, either a person or a thing, or a type of work, are written as two words.

    behavior analyst   metal work
    iron worker   needle carrier
    lens cutting

Exceptions: proofreader, proofreading, pacemaker

2. Letters (designating shape or use with special significance) need not be joined with a hyphen to a following noun.

    beta streptococci   X zone
    T tube   Y incision

Exception: x-ray

3. Compounds formed with "end," "back" or "side" are written as two words.

    back passage   end results
    back pressure   side arm
    end organ   side effects
    end picture   side passage

Exception: background

4. Compounds formed with "after" are hyphenated.

    after-effects   after-treatment

5. When "over" and "under" indicate degree, they are joined

without a hyphen; when they indicate position, they are used as separate words.

> overexcitement under side
> overstimulate under surface
> undernourished

6. "Cross" is used as an adjective or adverb and is not joined to a following word.

> cross immunization cross passage
> cross immunize cross section

7. Combinations of "self" with a following word are not hyphenated unless they are used as compound adjectives preceding nouns.

> self adjusting self respect
> self evident self-adjusting bandage

8. "Pseudo" and "quasi" are considered as prefixes and are joined to single words without a hyphen. Before compound words they should be used as adjectives.

> pseudo diabetes insipidus
> pseudoxanthoma
> quasipsychiatric

9. Nouns and adjectives ending in "up" are hyphenated; verbs are written as two words.

> A follow-up examination was made
> A flare-up occurred
> We followed up the evidence

Exceptions: makeup, setup

10. The suffix "like" is joined without a hyphen when it follows a mono-syllable (except one ending in "l") but takes a hyphen when it follows a polysyllable or a monosyllable ending in "l."

> conelike
> endothelium-like
> roll-like

11. "Counter" should be joined to a following single word without a hyphen whenever it can be so written without producing an awkward compound. When it is used with a hyphenated

or a two-word compound or with a phrase, it should be used as a separate adjective or adverb.

>   counteract
>   counterextension
>   counterincision
>   counter reverberations (to avoid doubling the "r")
>   counter spinal punctures

12. "Fold" should be joined without a hyphen to a numeral consisting of one word and used as a separate word when the numeral is composed of two or more words.

>   twofold   a thousandfold
>   twentyfold   one hundred fold
>   twenty-four fold   four thousand fold
>   a hundredfold

Proper names used adjectivally are not changed from their original form, as in "Argyll Robertson pupil" (named from Douglas Argyll Robertson) and "Brown-Séquard sign" (named from Charles Edouard Brown-Séquard). The "Binet-Simon test" is named from Binet and Simon, two investigators. Although it is proper to hyphenate such a combination of two names when they are used as a unit modifier, they should be joined with "and" when they are used as nouns: "the Pels-Macht test," but "the test of Pels and Macht."

Following is a list of preferred word combinations. When compounds similar to those in this list are encountered, they should be treated analogously.

Adams-Stokes (adj.)	bacillus carrier	blood stream
after-treatment	barbers' itch	blood vessel
air passage	base line	bloodletting
airplane	bedridden	bone ash
airway	bedtime	borderline
amino acid	belles-lettres	bow leg
amino nitrogen	Bence Jones	Braxton Hicks
aminoacetic acid	beta streptococci	breast feeding
ankle drop	bile duct	breast milk
Argyll Robertson	Binet-Simon (adj.)	brewers' yeast
arm band	birth rate	Brown-Séquard
athlete's foot	black-out	cannot
autointoxication	blindspot	carbolfuchsin
axis-cylinder	blindworm	

92 *Medical Writing*

carbon dioxide–combining power
case reports
Cheyne-Stokes (adj.)
chickenpox
childbirth
cleancut
clubfoot
coconut
cod liver oil
cogwheel
color blindness
contraindicate
corn starch
cottonseed oil
courthouse
cover glass
cover slip
co-worker
cow's milk
cowpox
cracker meal
cream-colored
cresyl blue
cross section
daylight
downhill (adj. & adv.)
dyestuff
ear drum
ear phone
editor in chief
end result
erythema exudativum
everyday (adj.)
ex-president
eyeball
eyeground
far sight
feebleminded
feedback
fellow men
fellow workers
finger nail
finger tip
fingerbreadth

firsthand
flatfoot
fluidounce
fluidrachm
foodstuff
foolproof
foot and mouth disease
foot candle
foot drop
footplate
forearm
foreleg
forelimb
forequarter
forward-most
fowlpox
fresh air camp
frostbite
full-fledged
full term (adj.)
gallbladder
gallstone
gastrointestinal
glassblowers' cataract
goldfish
gram-negative
gram-variable
guniea pig
gutta-percha
hair line
halfway
hang-over
harelip
hat band
hay fever
head piece
head rest
heart block
high school pupil
hindleg
hindlimb
hindquarter
horse serum
hourglass

housemaid's knee
housework
hydrogen ion concentration
hypoacidity
ice bag
ice box
ice pack
ice water
ill health
infrared
intragroup
iron deficiency state
isamine blue
jawbone
joint disease
keynote
knee joint
knock knee
lactic acid bacillus
lantern slide
life-termer
lip rouge
lipstick
live stock
long-continued (adj.)
loud speaker
lunchroom
lymph nodes
makeup
man power
medicolegal
meter candle
methylene blue
micromeasurements
micromethod
microorganism
midbrain
midline
milliampere minute
millicurie hours
milligram hour
mother's milk
motion picture
motorcar

Spelling

mouth piece	post mortem (other constructions)	subject matter
nationwide		sum total
near point	postoffice	sun bath
near sight	postoperative	surgeon general
nearby (adj.)	printers' ink	swimmers' itch
nerve head	privatdozent	symptom complex
new growth	product-moment method	test tube
newborn		textbook
no one	pulse rate	to wit
nose clip	quicksilver	today
nose piece	radioactivity	toe drop
olive oil	rat bite fever	toe nail
oneself	Rh factor (when it does not precede a noun)	tomorrow
openmindedness		tongue-tie
operating room		tonight
orang-utan	roundworm	transatlantic
osteoid-osteoma	safety pin	trypan blue
outdoors	Samoa pox	tsetse fly
outpatient	sand fly	tuning fork
over-all	school children	twenty odd
overfeeding	seesaw	twofold
overnight (adj. & adv.)	setup	ultraviolet
	sheep pox	un-American
pacemaker	shellfish	vice president
pansinusitis	short circuit	wartime (adj.)
past pointing	short-cut (adj. & v.)	water supply
per cent	short cut (n.)	wavelength
per cent hour	shotgun	well-being
pinhead	sickroom	wetnurse
pinpoint	smallpox	whipworm
pinprick	so-called	whooping cough
poison ivy	so far as	widespread
poppyseed oil	sometime*	worldwide
postcard	split pea	worth while
postmortem (adj. preceding noun)	standpoint	wrist drop
	stillborn	wryneck
	stopcock	
	stopwatch	

Use of Hyphens in Compound Adjective Modifiers

As has been said, hyphens are not necessary when the meaning is clear without them. The principles to be set forth here are

---
*Often must be two words.

generally followed in medical periodicals, exceptions being made only when misunderstanding or confusion might arise. The tendency is toward elimination of unnecessary hyphens.

When one of the elements of a compound adjective contains more than one word, the adjectives should be connected by a hyphen and an en dash should connect the compound adjective with the noun. An example is "blood-sugar–regulating mechanism." Such a complicated combination should be avoided whenever possible.

The following types of compound adjectives require hyphens:

1. Combinations of an adverb modifying an adjective or a participle.

>   well-established principles
>   ill-defined methods
>   an almost-cured lesion
>   a seldom-performed operation
>   the best-known book
>   little-stressed complications
>   far-reaching consequences
>   less-evident manifestations
>   ever-increasing importance
>   so-called

2. Combinations of an adjective and a noun.

>   connective-tissue changes
>   full-term infant
>   present-day practice
>   prickle-cell layer
>   slit-lamp examination
>   dark-field examination
>   low-grade fever
>   hanging-drop culture
>   old-time customs
>   round-cell sarcoma
>   wet-ashing method

3. Combinations of a noun modifier and a noun.

>   slide-precipitation test
>   complement-fixation test
>   roentgen-ray dermatitis
>   bone-conduction time
>   dextrose-tolerance tests

blood-sugar values
bundle-branch block

4. Combinations of a cardinal numeral and a noun.

one-day period
a 2-day-old boy
a two-stage operation
a two-platform method
two-point discrimination
a 14-week fetus

5. Combinations of an ordinal numeral and a noun.

second-grade pupils
third-grade material
a third-stage operation
first-class methods

6. Combinations in which the name of a color is modified by a descriptive noun or by an adjective, either descriptive or denoting a secondary color. (A hyphen is needed, however, when two coordinate adjectives of color are used—see paragraph 10, page 86.)

bluish-red lesions
olive-green lesions
deep-blue lesions
slate-blue lesions
silvery-white lesions
crystal-white lesions

7. Miscellaneous, more complicated combinations.

end-to-end anastomosis
a side-to-side connection
up-to-date methods

8. Combinations in which a noun is used as the object of the present participle of a transitive verb.

habit-forming drugs
skin-sensitizing substances
blood-sugar–regulating mechanism
blood-coagulating medium

9. Combinations of a participle with an adverb or a preposition.

heaped-up tissue
broken-off ends

10. Combinations of a noun and a participle.
> a breast-fed infant
> a dark-adapted eye
> time-honored traditions
> formaldehyde-fixed tissue

11. Combinations of "first" or "last" or an ordinal numeral with a participle.
> the last-mentioned author
> the first-published article
> the first-removed suture
> the third-born child

12. Combinations of "long" and a participle.
> long-standing tuberculosis
> long-established customs
> a long-continued discharge
> long-maintained remissions

13. Combinations of two nouns used coordinately to modify another noun.
> calcium-phosphorus ratio
> the Binet-Simon test

14. Combinations of two adjectives used coordinately to modify a noun.
> toxic-infectious dystrophy
> manic-depressive psychosis

15. Combinations of two adjectives or a noun and an adjective to modify a noun.
> tenth-normal hydrochloric acid
> all-important principles
> stony-hard lesions
> species-specific reactions
> water-resistant fabric
> Wassermann-fast serum

16. Combinations of an adjective and a participle.
> full-grown rabbits
> double-nucleated cell
> broad-shouldered men
> American-born children
> medium-sized papules
> normal-looking skin

  Exception: newborn infant

17. Combinations of a preposition and a noun.
> before-treatment tests

The following combinations should be hyphenated in any construction in which they occur:

1. Combinations of two coordinate adjectives.
> The psychosis was considered to be manic-depressive.

2. Combinations of two coordinate nouns or adjectives of color.
> The skin was blue-black.

VARIANT ENDINGS OF ADJECTIVES

One of the reforms in spelling adopted by many medical publications is the elimination of the "al" ending on adjectives. This reform was first strongly emphasized by Dr. George M. Gould,[3] in 1896.

> The incongruities of medical nomenclature," he said, "and the stock-still standing of irrational conservatism lead one to wonder if we are ever to awaken to the need of phiologic civilization.
>
> One of my four kind critics once wrote me remonstrating, solely on the ground of euphony, against cutting the *al* off the tail end of adjectives. . . . Either one thing or the other; if you refuse to say *chemic* and *theoretic,* then you must not say *scientific* and *hydrochloric.* If you make us say *chemical* and *theoretical,* then, like a sucking dove we will roar you for *consistency* and ask that you be *scientifical,* or else we will prescribe *nitrical* and *hydrochlorical* acid for your alarming *gastrical* torpor and obstinacy.

Dr. Gould submitted the following alarming example of the effects of carrying the "al" ending to extremes:

> SOME SCIENTIFIC DIFFICULTIES. The patient was . . . ascitical and cyanotical . . . had an anemical (dicrotical or anacrotical) murmur; splanchnical and splenical dullness was pronounced. Neither the allopathical nor the homeopathical consultants could determine whether the affection was of extrinsical or intrinsical origin, whether anabolical, katabolical, atrophical, septicemical, lithemical, leutical, hemical, hemolytical, thermical, tabetical, hepatical or encephalical. The specialists were called in, and laryngoscopical, ophthalmoscopical, gynecological and otoscopical examinations were made. The laryngoscopical man said a diphtheritical membrane was forming, and the

---
[3]Gould, G. M.: Concerning medical language. *J. A. M. A.*, 26:1007, May 23, 1896.

phrenical nerve was pressed upon. The next averred the difficulty was esophorical or exophorical, that a blenorrhagical inflammation, perhaps a rheumatical iritis, existed. After an endoscopical examination the gynecological expert said pelvical (or pubical) disorder was present, and a bad cystical, spermatical and chorionical state of affairs. The ear-man claimed that the disease was specifical, that the otical ganglion was syphilitical and its condition pathognomonical. The diagnostical and prognostical difficulties were certes becoming most prolifical!

As to therapeutical measures, one advised cardiacal and tonical treatment, another hypodermical; one thought hydriatical methods good, another antiphlogistical, while still another suggested hyponotical and soporifical agents. Galvanical and faradical electricity, as well as statical and franklinical, were advised. The surgeon after a diagnostical incision (under anesthetical precautions) spoke of a plastical operation. Caustical applications to the throat were considered good, and the exhibition of prussical, or of borical, nitrical and hydrochlorical acids, perhaps also carbolical with malical and acetical acid drinks. The general physician thought antineuralgical and antirheumatical prescriptions sufficient, but the obstetrician would have added oxytocical ones.

The patient died of alcoholical paretical dementia, superinduced, it is thought, by despair at the orthographical and phonetical conservatism of progressive Americans.

The following list of adjectives with variant endings indicates a trend in modern usage. I consider the "ic" ending preferable in practically all medical words.[4] (Italics have been used to indicate exceptions to this general practice and variations in meaning.)

aeronautic	anthropometric	chronologic
alphabetic (pertaining to an alphabet)	*arithmetical*	classic (typical)
	astronomic	*classical* (pertaining to classical civilization and languages)
	atypical	
alphabetical (in the order of the letters of the alphabet)	bacteriologic	
	biochemical	
	biographic	*clinical*
	biologic	criminologic
analytic	botanic	cylindric
anatomic	bronchoscopic	cytologic
anthropologic	*chemical*	dermatologic

[4]It will be noted that for a few words in the list two endings and two meanings are indicated. An interesting discussion of such distinctions is given by H. W. Fowler (*A Dictionary or Modern English Usage*. Oxford, Clarendon Press. 1930, p. 249, article on "-ic(al)") .

dynamic
economic (pertaining to economics
economical (thrifty)
elliptic
embryologic
empiric
endemic
entomologic
epidemic
epidemiologic
ethnographic
etiologic
etymologic
galenic (*galenical* is the noun)
genealogic
generic
geographic
geometric
gonococcic
gynecologic
hemianopic
histologic
historic (celebrated in history)
historical (relating to history)
hypodermic
hypothetic
hysterical
immunologic

logical
macroscopic
magic (pertaining to magic)
magical (resembling the effects of magic)
meteorologic
methodical
microscopic
morphologic
mystic
neurologic
nosologic
obstetric
ophthalmologic
optic (pertaining to the eye)
optical (pertaining to light or to the science of optics)
otolaryngologic
paradoxic
parasitic
parasitologic
parenthetic*
pathogenic
pathognomonic
pathologic
pediatric
periodic

pharmaceutic (drugs)
pharmaceutical (pharmacy)
pharmacologic
philosophic
physiologic
problematic
psychiatric
psychic
psychologic
rhinologic
rhythmic
roentgenologic
serologic
sociologic
spheric (pertaining to the heavenly bodies)
spherical (sphere shaped)
staphylococcic
statistical
streptococcic
symmetric
teleologic
theoretic
therapeutic
topical
topographic
toxicologic
typographic
zoologic

POSSESSIVE WITH PROPER NAMES

The use of the possessive case with the names of physicians associated with diseases, tests and other entities frequently creates a problem. The solution may be simplified if the question is con-

*Except in the sense of "full of or addicted to the use of parentheses," in which "parenthetical" should be used.

sidered as one of logical English usage rather than as one involving a set form for each phrase. In general, the use of the possessive form relates the thing designated to the worker for whom it is named more emphatically and personally than does the use of the name as an adjective modifier.

The following list gives examples of correct usage:

> Wassermann's test became popular.
> The Wassermann test is widely used.
> A Wassermann test was made.
> Three Wassermann tests were made.
> Wassermann tests are made daily.
> Ewing's sarcoma was described in detail.
> The Ewing sarcoma is one of the important types.
> A Ewing tumor was found.
> Six Ewing tumors were studied.
> Parkinson's disease is well known.
> The man had Gaucher's disease.
> Flexner's dysentery is different from Sonne's.
> Flexner dysentery was prevalent in that country.
> The Betz cell is distinctive.
> Betz cells were observed.
> Examination showed numerous Hassall corpuscles.
> Meckel's diverticulum is present in some persons.
> Bence Jones protein was present.
> The patient had Argyll Robertson pupils.
> The Argyll Robertson pupil is unmistakable.
> He had Hutchinson teeth.
> Shive's solution is prepared as follows:
> Shive's solution (or Shive solution) was used.
> The Masson stain was employed.
> Masson's stain is easily prepared.
> He took some Masson stain.

It will be noted that with an article, direct or indirect, the possessive form is not used, with the name becoming a noun used as an adjective modifier. In instances in which an article is not used, the possessive form may or may not be employed, depending on the degree of personal relationship or possessiveness, and the emphasis that one wishes to express.

In instances in which two names joined with a hyphen are used as a modifier, the possessive form should never be used.

> Niemann-Pick disease

the Prausnitz-Küstner phenomenon
a Binet-Simon test
Hand-Schüller-Christian disease

Possessive of Names Ending in a Sibilant

The possessive of a word of more than one syllable which ends in "s" or in some other sibilant is regularly formed by the addition of an apostrophe. When a word ends in "ce," however, or when the final sibilant is silent, an apostrophe followed by "s" is added.

Hippocrates' writings   Horace's odes
Collins' method   Bourgeois's works

To form the possessive of a monosyllable, an apostrophe followed by "s" is added.

Bass's sign   Wise's comments

CLASSICAL TERMINOLOGY

Medical words are derived almost entirely from Latin and Greek, often from Greek through latinized forms. Errors in medical writing are frequently seen in the use of plurals of classical nouns and in the terminations of modifying adjectives in accordance with number and gender.

As stated earlier in this book, the use of English names for diseases and anatomic structures is desirable. If, however, an author wishes to use the classical terms he should be careful to see that the forms are correct and should use anatomic names adopted by the BNA.

Diphthongs

When Latin or Greek words have been taken into the English language, diphthongs need not be retained, and in the publications of the American Medical Association such words are written without diphthongs—e.g. hemorrhage, anemia, polycythemia. Diphthongs are not used in Latin names of diseases. They are used in names of microorganisms when these names have been officially adopted by scientific societies.

The diphthongs "ae" and "oe" should be written with separate letters in Latin and in German words, and in English words derived from Latin or from Greek through Latin when these words retain the diphthong. The ligatures "ae" and "oe" should be used in Old English, in French and in some other modern languages.

Plurals

English plurals should be used whenever available, except, of course, when they are followed by Latin or Greek modifiers. English plurals should be employed for the names of organisms used as common nouns whenever they can be formed easily (amebas, spirochetes, uncinarias, rickettsias; but streptococci and staphylococci). All names ending in "a" are given English plurals except those in the accompanying list of classical plurals as yet retained.

The plural of the Latin neuter word "punctum" (a point) is "puncta," though it is not infrequently misspelled "punctae" as if feminine.

The following plural forms are recommended:

ACCEPTED ENGLISH PLURALS

abscissas	craniums	glomuses
acetabulums	curriculums	gummas
amebas	deliriums	gymnasiums
anlages	dictums	hematomas
antrums	duodenums	hernias
aortas	endotheliomas	indexes
apexes	enemas	inoculums
appendixes	epitheliomas	lacunas
areolas	erythemas	lamellas
auras	exanthems	laminas
axillas	femurs	lipomas
cannulas	fetuses	lumens
carcinomas	fibromas	maculas
chondromas	fibulas	maxillas
cochleas	fistulas	meatuses
collyriums	foramens	mediums (expect for "media" of eye)
comedos	formulas	
condylomas	foveas	
conjunctivas	ganglions*	meniscuses
corneas	glaucomas	microns

*In the *Archives of Neurology and Psychiatry* the plural "ganglia" is used.

Spelling

ACCEPTED ENGLISH PLURALS

myceliums	pterygiums	sputums
myomas	radiuses	stigmas
myxomas	retinas	stomas
nebulas	sanatoriums	stromas
ostiums	sarcomas	syllabuses
patellas	scapulas	symposiums
perineums	scleras	synechias
plasmas	scotomas	tibias
plexuses	septums	traumas
polyps (plural of polyp)	sequestrums	tympanums
	serums	ulnas
primiparas	solariums	uveas
psammomas	spectrums	vaginas

FOREIGN PLURALS AS YET RETAINED

alveoli	fundi	polypi (plural of polypus)
ampullae	hili	
apparatus	humeri	protozoa
bacteria	larvae	puncta
bronchi	maxima	quanta
calices	media (of eye)	rami
cortices	minima	rugae
criteria	nevi	sarcinae
data	nidi	sequelae (plural of sequela)
desiderata	nuclei	
diverticula	ova	spermatozoa
dorsa	papillae	striae
emboli	pelves	uteri
fenestrae	phenomena	verrucae
fibrillae	plasmodia	vertebrae
foci	pleurae	viscera
fossae		

Terminations

Terminations of classical nouns and adjectives are often used incorrectly. The following table shows the gender of certain nouns according to termination, and these may serve as prototypes:

GENDER OF NOUNS ACCORDING TO TERMINATIONS

Masculine	*Feminine*	*Neuter*
US second declension, lupus, nevus	IS psoriasis, dermatitis	US third declension, ulcus,

GENDER OF NOUNS ACCORDING TO TERMINATIONS

Masculine	Feminine	Neuter
	A tinea, verruca— except hydroa and words ending in MA	corpus MA sarcoma, erythema, chloasma
ES herpes	AS callositas, fragilitas	AS erysipelas
	IES scabies, canities	
EN lichen	E acne	UM molluscum
		U cornu
		EN sudamen
X anthrax	X cicatrix, pompholyx	
ER zoster		
IO pernio		
DO comedo	DO livedo	ON epidermophyton, kerion
	GO impetigo, vitiligo	

The greatest source of error is provided by words ending in "a." All words that end in "a" in the singular are feminine except for "hydroa" and those ending in "ma," which are neuter: e.g. hydroa aestival*e*, hydroa gravidar*um*, erythema bullos*um*, chloasma uterin*um*, xeroderma pigmentos*um*. "Verruca" is often a stumbling block, though according to the rule it is obviously a feminine noun and thus requires a feminine adjective, as verruca plan*a*.

Mistakes are constantly made in the words *"Spirochaeta"* (feminine) and *"Treponema"* (neuter). The correct uses of these words with the adjectives "pallidus, -a, -um" and "pertenuis, -is, -e" are *"Spirochaeta pallida"* and *"Spirochaeta pertenuis," "Treponema pallidum"* and *"Treponema pertenue."*

Latin words of the second declension ending in "us," such as lup*us* erythematos*us*, are masculine, whereas words of the third declension ending in "us," such as ulc*us* moll*e* and corp*us* lute*um*, are neuter.

Nouns ending in "is," with a few unimportant exceptions, are feminine. Examples are dermatit*is* factiti*a*, neurit*is* nodos*a* and arthrit*is* fungos*a*.

"Callositas" is a feminine noun, but "erysipelas" is neuter. Fortunately, these words seldom are followed by qualifying adjectives.

Glaring errors which occur frequently in medical writing concern the comparative forms of the words "magnus" (large) and "parvus" (small). The comparative forms are, respectively, "major" and "minor," which are declined in the nominative as follows:

	Masculine	Feminine	Neuter
SINGULAR	major	major	majus
PLURAL	majores	majores	majora
SINGULAR	minor	minor	minus
PLURAL	minores	minores	minora

The correct term designating the large lip of the vulva is "labi*um* maj*or*," and for the smaller lip, "labi*um* min*us*"; in regard to these, mistakes are rarely made.

Errors are found at times in speaking of a lesion which is unilateral. The expression "unius lateralis" is incorrect. Either the adjective "unilateralis" or the two words "unius lateris" may be used, "unius" being the genitive singular of the adjective "unus, -a, -um" and "lateris" the genitive singular of the noun "latus" (nevus unilateralis, nevus unius lateris).

For further information on classical terminology the reader is referred to an article by the late Dr. Howard Fox.[5]

---

[5] Fox, Howard: Common errors in dermatologic terminology. *Arch. Dermat. Syph.*, 7:499-504, April 1923.

7
CAPITALIZATION

Periodicals vary in their use of capitalization. The following principles represent some of the present trends in this matter.

Use capitals for:
1. The first word of a sentence, of course, as well as a complete sentence that is quoted directly, even when it occurs within another sentence.
2. The first word after a colon if it introduces a complete sentence.
3. The initial letters of words in headings, except for conjunctions, articles and short prepositions.
4. Proper names and titles, also adjectives derived from them unless they have acquired a special meaning.
5. Cited titles of books and articles in text (but see pages 120-129 for style in footnotes and bibliographies).
6. The latinized name of a person used in the genitive case (fissura Rolandi; ductus Botalli), except in the scientific name of an organism.
7. The names of phylums, classes, orders, families and genera, when referring to the scientific classification of organisms.
8. Proprietary and trademarked names.
9. The initial letter of the symbol of an element (Ca, Hg).

Write in lower case:
1. The first word of a fragmentary quotation (he urged "listening with the third ear").
2. The first word after a colon if it introduces a clause or list (not a complete sentence).

3. Those derivatives of proper nouns which have acquired an independent specialized meaning (bunsen burner; cesarean section; prussian blue; achilles tendon).
4. Species names, even those derived from proper nouns *(Sporotrichum beurmanni);* classes, orders, families, and genera when used to designate individual members (an arthropod, spirochetes of this type).
5. Generic names of drugs (penicillin, chloropropane).
6. Names of chemical elements or compounds when spelled out in full.

Write in capitals:	*Write in lower case:*
World War II, Civil War	the last great war
Federal Food, Drug and Cosmetic Act	a narcotic act was passed
Hippocratic oath	facies hippocratica, hippocratic finger
the Harvey Lecture	Graduate Fortnight lectures
Southern states	in southern regions
Chicago Medical Society	the various medical societies
North, South, East, West (when they refer to geographic divisions)	north, south, east, west (when they refer to direction)
Christian Science, Christian Scientist	Dr. Schweitzer, the Christian scientist and musicologist
Vienna School of Medicine	surgeons of the Vienna school
New York City	in the city of Chicago
Gram, Roentgen, as proper names	gram-negative, roentgen rays
Congress (United States)	an international congress

8
ABBREVIATIONS

IN SCIENTIFIC WRITING, abbreviations should be kept to a minimum and should follow a recognized standard. If nonstandard or special abbreviations must be employed, as in tabular or other condensed material, they should be explained in a footnote.

ADDRESSES

The following list gives standard abbreviations of the United States Government Printing Office for the states of the Union and for certain of its territories and possessions:

Ala.	Ga.	Miss.	N.Y.	Va.
Ariz.	Ill.	Mo.	Okla.	Vt.
Ark.	Ind.	Mont.	Oreg.	V.I.
Calif.	Kans.	N.C.	Pa.	Wash.
Colo.	Ky.	N.Dak.	P.R.	Wis.
Conn.	La.	Nebr.	R.I.	W.Va.
C.Z.	Mass.	Nev.	S.C.	Wyo.
D.C.	Md.	N.H.	S.Dak.	
Del.	Mich.	N.J.	Tenn.	
Fla.	Minn.	N.Mex.	Texas	

As a general rule, the names of states which contain only four or five letters should be spelled out (Idaho, Iowa, Maine, Ohio and Utah). The names of the other states are abbreviated when they follow the name of a city or county but not when they are used alone (in Cook County, Ill.; in Paterson, N.J.; in Kentucky).

The names of territories and possessions of the United States other than those listed should not be abbreviated.

It is usually not necessary to mention the state after the names of the following large cities:

Abbreviations

Baltimore	Denver	New Orleans	St. Paul
Boston	Detroit	New York	Salt Lake City
Brooklyn	Indianapolis	Oklahoma City	San Francisco
Buffalo	Iowa City	Omaha	Seattle
Chicago	Los Angeles	Philadelphia	
Cincinnati	Milwaukee	Pittsburgh	
Cleveland	Minneapolis	St. Louis	

When a Canadian city is mentioned, both the name of the province (written in full) and "Canada" should follow the name. (Exception: For Montreal, Toronto and Quebec the name of the province may be omitted.)

The name of a foreign country should never be abbreviated. The name of the country should be mentioned after the name of a foreign city unless it is clear from the text what country is concerned.

Before a name "Saint" is abbreviated (St. Louis, St. Paul). "Fort," "Mount" and "Santa" or "San," however, are not abbreviated (Fort Duquesne, Mount Vernon, Santa Barbara, San Francisco).

Street Addresses

In ordinary text matter, at the end of an article, and in general wherever space permits, street addresses should be written out in full. When abbreviation is necessary, the following forms are used:

441 Vine St.
80 N. Grand Blvd.
50 W. 50th Ave.
5 Bay State Rd.
601 Fullerton Parkway

302–1st Ave.
227–16th St.
501–1st St. N.W.
16th and P Sts.
1500 Medical Arts Bldg.

When a mailing address which includes a postal zip code number is cited, no comma is used after the name of the state, but the names of the city and state are separated by a comma: Pittsburgh, Pa. 15237.

Foreign Addresses

Foreign Addresses

66 Boulevard Saint-Michel, Paris, 6e, France
2 Rue Casimir-Delavigne, Paris, 6e, France

Sternwartenstrasse 8, Leipzig, C. 1, Germany
Rambler de Cataluña 72, Barcelona, Spain
Calle de Villarroel 17, Barcelona, Spain
Via Farini 6, Bologna, Italy
9 Wimpole St., London, W. 1, England
Mexico, D.F., Mexico

NAMES OF PERSONS

No abbreviations except the initials should be used for the names of persons (Thomas E. Clark or T. E. Clark, not Thos. E. Clark; Charles E. McFarlane or C. E. McFarlane, not Chas. E. McFarlane).

Titles and Degrees

One should never spell out "Mr.," "Mrs." or "Dr." before a proper name. "Major" should never be abbreviated. Other titles are abbreviated when they are used before the first name or initials but written in full when used before the family name alone:

Prof. A. T. Reed	Pres. M. A. Brown	Capt. Charles Ryerson
Professor Walton	President Eisenhower	Lieutenant Myerson
Supt. J. A. Milton	Major C. A. Wright	Dr. Osler

Degrees and titles following names are abbreviated. In capital lines in headings, degrees are set in large and small capitals (PH.D.; PHG).

Most medical periodicals put degrees in the order of rank, with Doctor of Medicine taking precedence when an author holds that degree. For instance, one would write "Robert Clark, M.D., Ph.D., " but not "Robert Clark, M.A., M.D."

ABBREVIATIONS OF DEGREES AND FELLOWSHIPS

Bachelor of Arts; Master of Arts .... B.A. or A.B.; M.A. or A.M.
Bachelor of Laws .... B.L. or LL.B.
Bachelor of Medicine; Bachelor of Music .... B.M. or M.B.
Bachelor of Science; Master of Science ....
  B.S., B.Sc. or Sc.B.; M.S. or M.Sc.
Doctor of Comparative Medicine .... M.C.D.
Doctor of Dental Medicine; Doctor of Dental Surgery .. D.M.D.; D.D.S.
Doctor of Laws .... J.D. or LL.D.

Doctor of Letters .... Litt.D. or D.Litt.
Doctor of Medicine .... M.D.
Doctor of Osteopathy .... D.O.
Doctor of Philosophy .... Ph.D.
Doctor of Public Health .... D.P.H.
Doctor of Science .... D.Sc. or Sc.D.
Doctor of Veterinary Medicine; Surgery .... D.V.M.; D.V.S.
Fellow of the American College of Physicians .... F.A.C.P.
Fellow of the American College of Surgeons ................F.A.C.S.
Fellow of the American College of Dentists .... F.A.C.D.
Fellow of the College of American Pathologists .... F.C.A.P.
Fellow of the International College of Surgeons .... F.I.C.S.
Fellow of the Royal College of Physicians; of Edinburgh; of Ireland ..
 F.R.C.P.; F.R.C.P.E.; F.R.C.P.I.
Fellow of the Royal College of Science .... F.R.C.Sc.
Fellow of the Royal College of Surgeons; of Edinburgh, in Ireland ..
 F.R.C.S.; F.R.C.S.E.; F.R.C.S.I.
Fellow of the Royal Society .... F.R.S.
Fellow of the Royal Society, Canada; of Edinburgh . F.R.S.C.; F.R.S.E.
Graduate in Pharmacy .... Ph.G.
Licentiate of the Royal College of Physicians, London ..... L.R.C.P.
Licentiate of the Royal College of Surgeons, London ...... L.R.C.S.
Master of Surgery .... M.C. or M.Ch.

DATES

In the following list are given the standard abbreviations for the names of the months:

Jan.	Apr.	Oct.
Feb.	Aug.	Nov.
Mar.	Sept.	Dec.

No abbreviation is used for May, June or July. The names of the other months should be abbreviated in bibliographic references and when both the day and the year are given (Feb. 29, 1948).

Frequently in descriptions of cases or of experiments, several dates in the same year are mentioned consecutively. The year is usually included in the first date of the series but only the month and day thereafter until the year changes, as in the following passage:

> A man aged 60 was admitted to the hospital on Mar. 5, 1947. He was operated on on Mar. 25 and was dismissed on May 10. In June, 1948, he was readmitted.

"In 1947-1948" may be used to designate the year that includes part of both. "From 1946 to 1948" should be used instead of "1946-1948" in text matter.

WEIGHTS, MEASURES AND TIME

Units of measurement are abbreviated after numerals but not otherwise. Some publishers limit this rule to units of the metric system (except meter, liter, kilometer and microgram which preferably should not be abbreviated). A few other abbreviations are similarly treated: A.M., P.M., C, F, D, r. For example:

10 A.M.	in the morning; in the forenoon
7 P.M.	in the afternoon
50 r	measured in roentgens
3 cm	marked off in centimeters
4 kg	per kilogram
10 mg	in each milligram
120 mm	a few millimeters
98° F	the Fahrenheit scale
1 D	the unit was the diopter
40° C	the centigrade thermometer

Abbreviations of units of measure are used in the singular form only. The following abbreviations for units of the metric system are those recommended in the "Pharmacopeia of the United States":

M = meter	dl = deciliter	gm = gram
dm = decimeter	ml = milliliter	dg = decigram
cm = centimeter	cc = cubic centimeter	cg = centigram
mm = millimeter	cu mm = cubic millimeter	mg = milligram
kg = kilogram		

The following standard abbreviations are permitted by some publishers in tabular matter or formulas only:

Å	angstrom unit	ft	foot
ac	alternating current	gal	gallon
ax.	axis	hr	hour
cyl.	cylinder	in.	inch
dc	direct current	kv	kilovolt
d. v.	double vibration	kva	kilovolt ampere
dB	decibel	lb	pound
dr.	drachm	μ	microns

mμ	millimicrons	oz	ounce
ma	milliampere	p.d.	prism diopter, papilla diameter
ma-min	milliampere minute	pt	pint
mCi	millicurie	qt	quart
mc-hr	millicurie hour	sec	second
mEq	milliequivalent	2nd	second
mg-hr	milligram hour	3rd	third
min	minute	yd	yard
mo	month		

There is a tendency in some fields to drop the periods in many abbreviations, especially in abbreviated units of measurement.

ABBREVIATIONS PERMISSIBLE IN OPHTHALMOLOGY

Abbreviations of measurements of squint, especially in series of values are as follows:

HP .... hyperphoria
HT .... hypertropia (with L or R)
XT and ST .... exotropia and esotropia (with L or R)
Similar abbreviations

Some other general abbreviations are these:

△ .... prism diopters
f.c. .... foot candles
p.d. or P.D. .... papilla diameter
R.E. and L.E. .... right eye and left eye
D. .... diopters (with values)
sph. (for spherical) and cyl. (for cylindrical) in such expressions as "+ 1.25 D. sph." "− 2.00 D. cyl."

Omission of D. and perhaps the sph. and cyl. in refractions is as follows:

+ 1.25 sph. − 2.00 cyl., axis 90
    Or
+ 1.25 − 2.00, axis 90

"Near" is used alone in expressions like "accommodation for near was normal."

Perimetry is written "field for 3/300 white" or "field for white, 3/300."

MISCELLANEOUS ABBREVIATIONS

Day and days should never be abbreviated, even in tables.

Names of chemical elements should be abbreviated only in tabular matter and formulas. Chemical symbols are not followed by a period (Ca, Hg).

One writes "an angle of 45 degrees." Symbols may be used if the expressions are complex and recur frequently, as in "angles of 15° 30′ 15″ and 45° 6′." The symbol for degrees may be omitted in expressions of temperature; thus, one may write "100 F" and "39 C" rather than "100° F" and "39° C"[1] The word degree should be spelled out in expressions of latitude and longitude if minutes and seconds are not mentioned, as in the phrase "a difference of 3 degrees of latitude." In some expressions the word "degree" may be omitted as in "latitude 42 north." Write "8° 45′ 15″."

In tables both clock time and extent of time may be written in figures. The time 25 minutes and 16 seconds past 3 o'clock may be written "3:25:16"; a period of 14 hours, 45 minutes and 30 seconds may be written "14° 45′ 30″."

British money of the period before the decimal system was adopted, when set in figures, is expressed as follows: £23 7s. 3d.

American money is expressed as follows: $15; $20.42; 56 cents.

In tables, signs and abbreviations should be used in place of words as much as practicable. Use + and − for positive and negative; >, < and = for greater than, less than and equals; ♂ or ☐ for male and ♀ or ○ for female. The sign % may be used in tables, but not elsewhere.

In text matter, a reaction or degree of change should be expressed with words rather than with symbols (4 plus, positive, negative, plus-minus). In tables, symbols may be used as is most convenient in the individual instance.

The basal metabolic rate is expressed in text matter as "−5 per cent" or "+ 18 per cent."

---

[1] It is necessary, however, to speak of "a rise of 1 degree (F)." Body temperature should be expressed preferably according to the Fahrenheit scale. If it is given in centigrade degrees, the Fahrenheit equivalent should follow in parentheses.

Dimensions are given as "4 by 5 by 7 inches," not "4 × 5 × 7 inches."

In ordinary matter, expressions of dosage should be spelled out. Write "4 grains (0.25 gm) three times a day," not "gr iv., t. i. d."

Except where condensation is an object, as in tables, one should write "eighth-molar" or "tenth-normal," not "M/8," "decinormal" or "N/10." If it is desirable for some special reason to use the fraction, the slant (virgule) instead of the horizontal line should be used to separate the numerator and the denominator. At times, when large or complicated fractions are involved, it may be clearer to write "0.25 normal" or "0.03 normal." Multiples of normal should be expressed as "three times normal" rather than as "3/N."

The abbreviation for the expression 1 to 1,000 is 1:1,000. Either form may be used, according to the author's preference.

SCIENTIFIC NAMES OF ORGANISMS

Bacteria

After the name of a species has been given in full, as *"Treponema pallidum,"* the generic name should be abbreviated, as *"T. pallidum,"* throughout the paper.

This rule applies only to the *same genus*. For instance, after *Streptococcus fecalis* has been mentioned once, *"Str. fecalis"* is used; but if another genus name is then mentioned, *Streptococcus fecalis* must be written out the next time it appears.

In tables, abbreviations may be used if the full name is given in the text, either preceding or following the table. If some organisms are mentioned in the table which are not referred to in the text and the application of this rule would give the table an awkward appearance, it usually is better to write out all the names in the table. If there are only two or three organisms which are not mentioned in the text and they are species of a common genus, such as *Staphylococcus,* the abbreviation for which is unmistakable, or of a genus other species of which are mentioned so frequently in the text that there is no danger of confusion, the genus names may be abbreviated in the table.

A name should be written in full in the heading for an abstract or a report in a society transaction and also the first time it appears in the text. In society transactions, after a name has been given in full once in a report, it should be abbreviated throughout that report and the discussion thereon; if the same organism is mentioned in another report the name should again be written in full.

Fungi and Parasites

Names of organisms which are well known to physicians, such as *Epidermophyton* and *Taenia*, are subject to the rules that govern the abbreviation of names of bacteria. There are many names, however, both of genuses and of species, which do not yet appear in medical dictionaries. In most medical publications abbreviations are not used, as a rule, unless the name appears in *Blakiston's New Gould Medical Dictionary* or *Dorland's Illustrated Medical Dictionary* together with a definition. If some of the names mentioned in an article have usable abbreviations and others do not, it is well to spell out all the names in the article.

Other Generic Names

Names of plants, animals and insects should not be abbreviated.

MISCELLANEOUS RULES

The expression "Figure 1" should be spelled out in ordinary text matter. One may write "Fig. 1" in parentheses. When "Figure" is used at the beginning of a legend, it is spelled out and capitalized.

> The heart (Fig. 1) shows decided enlargement.
> The heart shows decided enlargement (see Fig. 1).
> Figure 1. Enlargement of the heart.

Write "fourth cervical" and "second lumbar," rather than "C IV" or "L 2," except in tabular matter.

"BCG" and "QRS" are written without spacing. "P-R," "S-7" and "RS-T" intervals are hyphenated.

"BAL" (British antilewisite) is used without periods or spacing.

"U.S.P.," "N.N.D.," "N.F." and "BNA" are written without regular spacing. These abbreviations may follow the name of a drug without the interposition of a comma.

Tuning forks are designated as follows: C-2, C-1, C, c-1, c-2, etc., capital letters being used for sounds below middle C and lower case letters for those above it.

Both in the text and in tabular matter, "no. 3" should be used rather than "number 3." Whenever possible, "no." should be omitted (communication 3; Jaeger's test type 1).

When "page 6" appears in the text, the word "page" should not be abbreviated.

Abbreviations used only in prescriptions (or occasionally in tables) are given in Chapter 10.

9
NUMBERS

NUMBERS APPEAR FREQUENTLY in scientific—especially in statistical—articles; it is sometimes difficult to determine when they should be spelled out and when put in figures. The American Medical Association Press has therefore adopted various general and specific rules governing such usage in its publications.

Numbers of patients, cases or, when considered analogously, animals or specimens should be put in figures. If "one" is used in an indefinite rather than in a numerical sense (for instance, if "a patient" might be substituted), it may be spelled out.

Numbers designating measurements should, in general, be put in figures.

Miscellaneous numbers, concerning which instructions are not included in the specific rules to be given, should be spelled out for the numbers one to nine; for 10 and above figures should be used.

> A hospital of 49 rooms was built.
> We examined three fingers.
> He had consulted four physicians.

If, however, in an individual article there are several large numbers of items of any one category—for instance, injections or hospitals—it is advisable to use figures for all the numbers in that group.

SPECIFIC RULES

Set in figures both whole numbers and fractions denoting:

1. Numbers of cases or patients or, when considered analogously, animals or specimens in text and in roman and italic sideheads when corresponding figures appear in the text.

2. Values for measurements, such as temperature, pulse rate, respiratory rate, blood count, specific gravity, age, weight, height, length, breadth, area, capacity, degrees, percentages and ratios. (The amount of a dose, as a measurement, is put in figures, but the number of doses is considered with the miscellaneous numbers in the paper and spelled out.)
3. Dates: Jan. 18, 1948; January 18.
4. Clock time: 7 A.M., 6:30 P.M., 15 minutes and 20 seconds past 4 P.M.
5. Sums of money: $250, $1.50, 75 cents, £15 8s. 3d.
6. In tabular matter and in the headings of tables, every number that can be so expressed.
7. Numbers indicating serial position: page 22, case 3, table 5, chapter 10, Figure 1; group 1, type IV, grade 2, cat 3 A, dog 1096 (note omission of comma).
8. Experimental and laboratory results which involve duration of time.
9. Numbers above nine representing length of time: for 30 minutes, after 10 hours, 15 minutes past 1 P.M., 18 years ago, a 24-hour culture.
10. Any one-digit number used in conjunction with a two-digit number: 8 to 12 cell layers.

Spell out:
1. Ordinal numbers: the eighth patient, on the tenth day, in the eighteenth century.
2. Numbers used as nouns or in an indefinite sense: in the nineties, per hundred, per thousand, by fifties, per hundred grams (but per 25 pounds).
3. Numbers of doses or injections, families, litters, cultures, determinations, chapters.
4. All numbers except those of four digits in titles or subtitles of articles, in titles of abstracts and in titles cited in footnotes.

Numbers are spelled out as follows:

one-half the patients (hyphenate where "of" is omitted)
half the patients
a third of the patients

three fourths of the patients
one-half hour
half an hour
a half-hour
two and a half hours
three and one-half hours
increased by two thirds
twenty-four
one hundred and twenty-six
twenty-eight hundred
two thousand, three hundred and sixty
one million, three thousand, five hundred and one

A fraction should be hyphenated when it is used as an adjective, as in the phrase "one-half hour," or when ambiguity might result without the hyphen; when it is used as a noun, the hyphen may be omitted.

MISCELLANEOUS EXAMPLES

3 drops, capsules, tablets
2 tablespoons; 2 teaspoons
3 disk diameters
4 fingerbreadths
1 erythema dose
½ erythema dose
1 skin unit
50 roentgens
2 unit skin doses
three doses of neoarsphenamine
eight injections of a bismuth preparation
temperature of 96° F
a rise of 1 degree (F)
4 plus (not four plus or + + + + except in tables)
The epithelium contained from 2 to 10 cell layers.
His diet included one apple twice a day and two glasses of water each morning and each afternoon.
a 6-month fetus; a 9-week fetus; a 10-day embryo
a 10 mm embryo
a 6-day-old child; a 10-hour-old boy; an 8-week-old girl; a 10-month-old child; a 30-year-old man
a six-week period
after six-weeks' treatment
after six-weeks of treatment

Numbers

1947–1948 (the year including parts of both)
1946 to 1948
1947 and 1948
6-year molars
6 pounds 8 ounces
3 feet 6 inches
She was six months pregnant.
The child was born one month prematurely.
a 24-hour culture
size 7-4A shoes
2nd
3rd
pneumococci of type III, the type V pneumococcus, *Pneumococcus* type I
per hundred cubic centimeters, per thousand grams[1], per 10 gm.[1]
in each hundred cubic centimeters[1] [or] in each 100 cc
in each 10 gm.
layers I to VI of the cortex
leads I, II and III[2] of the electrocardiogram
the T wave in lead I, T_3, the QRS complex in lead III[3]
6 gm is used
5 drops was given
radioactive phosphorus—P^{32}
the valence of a radical—PO_4

EQUIVALENT VALUES

Metric Equivalents

In scientific matter metric units are given first, followed in parentheses by values according to other systems. In some instances an exact equivalent is needed—for instance, when a small dose of a

---

[1]"Per hundred cubic centimeters" is written rather than "per 100 cc" because the latter phrase would be read "per *one hundred cubic centimeters,*" an idiom not likely to be encountered. "Per 10 gm" is clear, since the phrase can be read in only one way. Either "in each 100 gm" or "in each hundred grams" is idiomatically correct; consequently, either may be used, according to an author's preference.

[2]Most journals devoted to cardiology use "leads I, II and III." *The Journal of the American Medical Association* uses "leads 1, 2 and 3" because arabic numerals are preferred whenever possible.

[3]"The T wave in lead III" is perhaps preferable to "T_3." When many values are given, however, the shorter expression is convenient. It is advisable to be as consistent as possible within an article and not to jump unnecessarily from one form to the other.

drug or the thickness of a lens is concerned. In others, an approximate equivalent is preferable. The diameter of a cutaneous lesion measuring 2 inches should be expressed as "5 cm" rather than as "5.08 cm" One should consider the accuracy with which measurement of the thing under consideration could be made.

Centigrade measurements may be converted to Fahrenheit: multiply by 9, divide by 5 and add 32. Fahrenheit may be converted to centigrade: subtract 32, multiply by 5 and divide by 9.

In computing approximate equivalents, one should compute the exact equivalent to from one to three decimal places and then take the nearest approximate value, rather than multiply by an approximate value (such as 2.5 cm for 1 inch rather than 2.54 cm). Approximate equivalents for metric and apothecaries' systems may be found in many books.

The following tables give equivalent values that are frequently needed:

AVOIRDUPOIS WEIGHTS

Oz	Gm	Kg	Lb	Gm	Kg	Lb	Gm	Kg
1	28.35		61	27,669.11	27.7	131	59,420.55	59.4
2	56.70		62	28,122.70	28.1	132	59,874.14	59.9
3	85.05		63	28,576.30	28.6	133	60,327.73	60.3
4	113.40		64	29,029.89	29.0	134	60,781.33	60.8
5	141.75		65	29,483.48	29.5	135	61,234.92	61.2
6	170.10		66	29,937.07	29.9	136	61,688.51	61.7
Lb	Gm	Kg	67	30,390.66	30.4	137	62,142.10	62.1
¼	113.40	0.11	68	30,844.26	30.8	138	62,595.69	62.6
½	226.80	0.23	69	31,297.85	31.3	139	63,049.29	63.0
¾	340.19	0.34	70	31,751.44	31.8	140	63,502.88	63.5
1	453.59	0.5	71	32,205.03	32.2	141	63,956.47	64.0
2	907.18	0.9	72	32,658.62	32.7	142	64,410.06	64.4
3	1,360.77	1.3	73	33,112.21	33.1	143	64,863.65	64.9
4	1,814.37	1.8	74	33,565.81	33.6	144	65,317.25	65.3
5	2,267.96	2.3	75	34,019.40	34.0	145	65,770.84	65.8
6	2,721.55	2.7	76	34,472.99	34.5	146	66,224.43	66.2
7	3,175.14	3.2	77	34,926.58	34.9	147	66,678.02	66.7
8	3,628.73	3.6	78	35,380.18	35.4	148	67,131.62	67.1
9	4,082.33	4.1	79	35,833.77	35.8	149	67,585.21	67.6
10	4,535.92	4.5	80	36,287.36	36.3	150	68,038.80	68.0
11	4,989.51	5.0	81	36,740.95	36.7	151	68,492.39	68.5
12	5,443.10	5.4	82	37,194.54	37.2	152	68,945.98	68.9
13	5,896.69	5.9	83	37,648.14	37.6	153	69,399.58	69.4
14	6,350.29	6.4	84	38,101.73	38.1	154	69,853.17	69.9
15	6,803.88	6.8	85	38,555.32	38.6	155	70,306.76	70.3
16	7,257.47	7.3	86	39,008.91	39.0	156	70,760.35	70.8
17	7,711.06	7.7	87	39,462.50	39.5	157	71,213.94	71.2
18	8,164.65	8.2	88	39,916.10	39.9	158	71,667.53	71.7
19	8,618.25	8.6	89	40,369.69	40.4	159	72,121.13	72.1
20	9,071.84	9.1	90	40,823.28	40.8	160	72,574.72	72.6
21	9,525.43	9.5	91	41,276.87	41.3	161	73,028.31	73.0

Numbers

AVOIRDUPOIS WEIGHTS—(Continued)

Oz	Gm	Kg	Lb	Gm	Kg	Lb	Gm	Kg
22	9,979.02	10.0	92	41,730.46	41.7	162	73,481.90	73.5
23	10,432.61	10.4	93	42,184.05	42.2	163	73,935.50	74.0
24	10,886.21	10.9	94	42,637.65	42.6	164	74,389.09	74.4
25	11,339.80	11.3	95	43,091.24	43.1	165	74,842.68	74.8
26	11,793.39	11.8	96	43,544.83	43.5	166	75,296.27	75.3
27	12,246.98	12.2	97	43,998.42	44.0	167	75,749.86	75.7
28	12,700.57	12.7	98	44,452.01	44.5	168	76,203.46	76.2
29	13,154.17	13.2	99	44,905.61	44.9	169	76,657.05	76.7
30	13,607.76	13.6	100	45,359.20	45.4	170	77,110.64	77.1
31	14,061.35	14.1	101	45,812.79	45.8	171	77,564.23	77.6
32	14,514.94	14.5	102	46,266.38	46.3	172	78,017.82	78.0
33	14,968.53	15.0	103	46,719.97	46.7	173	78,471.42	78.5
34	15,422.13	15.4	104	47,173.57	47.2	174	78,925.01	78.9
35	15,875.72	15.9	105	47,627.16	47.6	175	79,378.60	79.4
36	16,329.31	16.3	106	48,080.75	48.1	176	79,832.19	79.8
37	16,782.90	16.8	107	48,534.34	48.5	177	80,285.78	80.3
38	17,236.49	17.2	108	48,987.93	49.0	178	80,739.38	80.7
39	17,690.09	17.7	109	49,441.53	49.4	179	81,192.97	81.2
40	18,143.68	18.1	110	49,895.12	49.9	180	81,646.56	81.6
41	18,597.27	18.6	111	50,348.71	50.3	181	82,100.15	82.1
42	19,050.86	19.1	112	50,802.30	50.8	182	82,553.74	82.6
43	19,504.45	19.5	113	51,255.89	51.3	183	83,007.34	83.0
44	19,958.05	20.0	114	51,709.49	51.7	184	83,460.93	83.5
45	20,411.64	20.4	115	52,163.08	52.1	185	83,914.52	83.9
46	20,865.23	20.9	116	52,616.67	52.6	186	84,368.11	84.4
47	21,318.82	21.3	117	53,070.26	53.1	187	84,821.70	84.8
48	21,772.41	21.8	118	53,523.85	53.5	188	85,275.30	85.3
49	22,226.01	22.2	119	53,977.45	54.0	189	85,728.89	85.7
50	22,679.60	22.7	120	54,431.04	54.4	190	86,182.48	86.2
51	23,133.19	23.1	121	54,884.63	54.9	191	86,636.07	86.6
52	23,586.78	23.6	122	55,338.22	55.3	192	87,089.66	87.1
53	24,040.37	24.0	123	55,791.81	55.8	193	87,543.26	87.5
54	24,493.97	24.5	124	56,245.41	56.2	194	87,996.85	88.0
55	24,947.56	24.9	125	56,699.00	56.7	195	88,450.44	88.5
56	25,401.15	25.4	126	57,152.59	57.2	196	88,904.03	88.9
57	25,854.74	25.9	127	57,606.18	57.6	197	89,357.62	89.4
58	26,308.33	26.3	128	58,059.77	58.1	198	89,811.22	89.8
59	26,761.93	26.8	129	58,513.37	58.5	199	90,264.81	90.3
60	27,215.52	27.2	130	58,966.96	59.0	200	90,718.40	90.7

1 short ton = 2,000 lb. = 90.72 Kg. = 0.9072 metric ton
1 long ton = 2,240 lb. = 118.18 kg. = 1.01605 metric tons
1 metric ton = 2,200 lb. = 1,000 Kg. = 1.1023 short tons
0.9842 long ton
40,000 short tons = 36,300 metric tons

APOTHECARIES' AND METRIC WEIGHTS

Grains	Gm	Grains	Gm	Grains	Gm	Grains	Gm
1	0.06	16	1.04	31	2.01	46	2.98
2	0.13	17	1.10	32	2.07	47	3.04
3	0.19	18	1.16	33	2.14	48	3.11
4	0.26	19	1.23	34	2.20	49	3.17
5	0.32	20	1.29	35	2.27	50	3.24
6	0.39	21	1.36	36	2.33	51	3.30
7	0.45	22	1.42	37	2.40	52	3.36
8	0.52	23	1.49	38	2.46	53	3.43

APOTHECARIES' AND METRIC WEIGHTS (Continued)

9	0.58	24	1.55	39	2.53	54	3.50
10	0.65	25	1.62	40	2.59	55	3.56
11	0.71	26	1.68	41	2.65	56	3.62
12	0.78	27	1.75	42	2.72	57	3.69
13	0.84	28	1.81	43	2.78	58	3.75
14	0.91	29	1.88	44	2.85	59	3.82
15	0.97	30	1.94	45	2.91	60	3.88

Drachms	Gm	Drachms	Gm	Drachms	Gm	Drachms	Gm
1	3.88	3	11.65	5	19.44	7	27.17
2	7.76	4	15.50	6	23.36	8	31.04

APOTHECARIES' AND METRIC MEASURES OF CAPACITY

Minims	Ml	Minims	Ml	Minims	Ml	Minims	Ml	Minims	Ml
1	0.06	13	0.80	25	1.54	37	2.28	49	3.02
2	0.12	14	0.86	26	1.60	38	2.34	50	3.08
3	0.18	15	0.92	27	1.66	39	2.40	51	3.14
4	0.25	16	0.99	28	1.73	40	2.46	52	3.20
5	0.31	17	1.05	29	1.79	41	2.53	53	3.27
6	0.37	18	1.11	30	1.85	42	2.59	54	3.33
7	0.43	19	1.17	31	1.91	43	2.65	55	3.39
8	0.49	20	1.23	32	1.97	44	2.71	56	3.45
9	0.55	21	1.29	33	2.03	45	2.77	57	3.51
10	0.61	22	1.36	34	2.09	46	2.83	58	3.57
11	0.67	23	1.42	35	2.16	47	2.90	59	2.63
12	0.74	24	1.48	36	2.22	48	2.96	60	3.70

1 teaspoon (tsp) = 4–5 ml   1 quart (qt) = 0.9463 liter (1,000 ml)
1 tablespoon (tbsp) = 15 ml   1 gallon (gal) = 3.78 liter
1 pint (pt) = 473 ml

MEASURES OF LENGTH

Ft	In	Cm	Ft	In	Cm	Ft	In	Cm
	¼	0.64	2	7	78.74	5	4	162.56
	½	1.27	2	8	81.28	5	5	165.10
	¾	1.91	2	9	83.82	5	6	167.64
	1	2.54	2	10	86.36	5	7	170.18
	2	5.08	2	11	88.90	5	8	172.72
	3	7.62	3	0	91.44	5	9	175.26
	4	10.16	3	1	93.98	5	10	177.80
	5	12.70	3	2	96.52	5	11	180.34
	6	15.24	3	3	99.06	6	0	182.88
	7	17.78	3	4	101.60	6	1	185.42
	8	20.32	3	5	104.14	6	2	187.96
	9	22.86	3	6	106.68	6	3	190.50
	10	25.40	3	7	109.22	6	4	193.04
	11	27.94	3	8	111.76	6	5	195.58
	12	30.48	3	9	114.30	6	6	198.12
1	1	33.02	3	10	116.84	6	7	200.66
1	2	35.56	3	11	119.38	6	8	203.20
1	3	38.10	4	0	121.92	6	9	205.74
1	4	40.64	4	1	124.46	6	10	208.28
1	5	43.18	4	2	127.00	6	11	210.82
1	6	45.72	4	3	129.54	7	0	213.36

MEASURES OF LENGTH (Continued)

1	7	48.26	4	4	132.08	7	1	215.90
1	8	50.80	4	5	134.62	7	2	218.44
1	9	53.34	4	6	137.16	7	3	220.98
1	10	55.88	4	7	139.70	7	4	223.52
1	11	58.42	4	8	142.24	7	5	226.06
2	0	60.96	4	9	144.78	7	6	228.60
2	1	63.50	4	10	147.30	7	7	231.14
2	2	66.04	4	11	149.86	7	8	233.68
2	3	68.58	5	0	152.40	7	9	236.22
2	4	71.12	5	1	154.94	7	10	238.76
2	5	73.66	5	2	157.48	7	11	241.30
2	6	76.20	5	3	160.02	8	0	243.84

1 ft = 0.3048 meter
10 ft = 3.048 meters
1,000 ft = 304.8 meters [or] 0.3 kilometer (km)
1 mile = 1.6093 km

MEASURES OF AREA

1 sq in = 6.4516 sq cm
1 sq ft = 0.0929 sq meter
1 sq yd = 0.8361 sq meter

MEASURES OF VOLUME

1 cu in = 16.387 cu cm
1 cu ft = 0.0283 cu meter
1 cu yd = 0.7646 cu meter

MEASURES OF CAPACITY

Fluidrachms	Ml	Liters	Fluidounces	Ml	Liters
1	3.7	0.004	1	29.57	0.03
2	7.39	0.007	2	59.15	0.06
3	11.09	0.011	3	88.72	0.09
4	14.79	0.015	4	118.29	0.12
5	18.48	0.018	5	147.87	0.15
6	22.18	0.022	6	177.44	0.18
7	25.88	0.026	7	207.02	0.21
8	29.57	0.030	8	236.59	0.24
			9	266.16	0.27
			10	295.73	0.30
			11	325.31	0.33
			12	354.88	0.35
			13	384.46	0.38
			14	414.03	0.41
			15	443.61	0.44
			16	473.18	0.47
			17	502.75	0.50
			18	532.33	0.53
			19	561.90	0.56
			20	591.47	0.59

ENUMERATIONS

In enumerations, periods follow arabic numerals which designate complete sentences, items in lists separated by periods and tabulated items. Parentheses are used around arabic numerals which designate clauses or listed items separated by commas or semicolons. An example of enumeration of complete sentences is given in Chapter 3, in the section on conclusions. Examples of other types of enumeration follow.

> The cases were grouped according to the result of treatment as follows:
> 1. Cases in which the result of treatment was favorable: tension normal; visual acuity 1/2 or more.
> 2. Cases in which the result of treatment was less favorable: tension normal; visual acuity from 1/60 to 1/3.
> 3. Cases in which the result of treatment was unfavorable: tension raised or visual acuity less than 1/60 or eye removed.
>
> There are three essential factors in the development of experimental cholesterol arteriosclerosis: (1) cholesterol in the diet, (2) hypercholesteremia and (3) injury to the intima of the arteries.

10
PHARMACEUTIC PRODUCTS AND PRESCRIPTIONS

IN MEDICAL WRITING, particularly that dealing with the treatment of disease, medicaments are mentioned frequently. Established products should be designated by the official English names given in the *Pharmacopeia of the United States*. The most accurate descriptive name available for a drug should be employed, and the exact chemical composition should be included. In the spelling of chemical terms it is well to follow the rules adopted by the American Chemical Society.

TRADEMARKED DRUGS

The names of trademarked drugs are usually capitalized or given in quotation marks. They may be quoted *in toto* the first time they are used—e.g., "Paredrine hydrobromide ophthalmic," "Paredrine hydrobromide aqueous"; after that, shortened forms such as "ophthalmic Paredrine" and "aqueous Paredrine" are used. When the initial capital is reserved for official preparations, the quotation marks are used to identify trade-marked products. Many publications now put a superior designation ® after the registered trade mark name of any preparation the first time that name is mentioned.

ENDOCRINE AND PHARMACEUTIC NOMENCLATURE

Progress in the use of endocrine preparations and of anti-infective agents has been so rapid that there is much confusion in the minds of physicians concerning the use of these preparations, their sources, potencies and identities. Unless correct nomenclature is used in medical writing and speaking, confusion will continue to exist.

Because the word "hormone" is all too often applied erroneously, it probably is best to avoid this term and use "endocrine substance," "principle" or "factor." It also is best to make reference whenever possible to the standardization of these preparations in terms of weight of the active components and not to units.

Other terms widely misapplied are "female sex hormone," "male sex hormone" and "corpus luteum hormone." They should be referred to as "estrogen," "androgen" and "progestin," and further defined according to their exact nature. Likewise, "thyroid extract" is commonly misused when the writer actually means desiccated thyroid. This is not an extract but simply the dried gland.

When sulfanilamide, sulfapyridine and sulfathiazole were introduced as therapeutic agents, the term "sulfa drugs" was born. There are few more meaningless words than "sulfa"; it has no scientific standing and should never be used, even in a popular sense. When a writer wishes to use a broadly descriptive word, reference should be made to "sulfonamide," a term that has meaning and is recognized as being reserved for this new class of chemotherapeutic agents.

Another word that has assumed almost household familiarity is "antibiotic." It is now reserved by the majority of physicians for extracts from substances such as molds, fungi and bacteria and is applied to drugs such as penicillin, streptomycin and tyrothricin. These three drugs have definitely different properties, and describing any one of them simply as an antibiotic would not provide any worthwhile information. There may even be reason to specify the type of penicillin under discussion.

PRESCRIPTIONS

So that prescriptions may appear properly in an article, they should be uniform in style and either wholly in Latin or wholly in English. The use of English is preferable. Many newer products do not have latinized endings. An example of a prescription in English is:

	Gm or Cc	
Magnesium oxide	10	ʒiiss
Bismuth subcarbonate	20	ʒv
Syrup of acacia, water; each in sufficient quantity		or
To make	200	ʒviii

Directions: Take 1 tablespoon as required after meals, plain or in water.

The same prescription in Latin would be:

℞ Magnesii oxidi	10	ʒiiss
Bismuthi subcarbonatis	20	ʒv
Syrupi acaciae	q.s.	or
Aquae destillatae	q.s.	
Ad	200	fl ʒ viii

M. Sig.: Take 1 tablespoon as required after meals, plain or in water.

In Latin prescriptions, certain words may be abbreviated:

caps. (capsula)	garg. (gargarisma)	pulv. (pulvis)
cerat. (ceratum)	gland. (glandula)	spt. (spiritus)
comp. (compositus)	glyc. (glyceritum)	suppos. (suppositorium)
conf. (confectio)	inf. (infusum)	syr. (syrupus)
cort. (cortex)	lin. (linimentum)	tr., tinct. (tinctura)
decoc. (decoctum)	liq. (liquor)	trit. (tritura)
elix. (elixir)	mist. (mistura)	troch. (trochiscus)
emp. (emplastrum)	ol (oleum)	ung. (unguentum)
enem. (enema)	pil (pilula)	vin. (vinum)
fldxt. (fluidextractum)		

It is well to avoid abbreviating the names of the drugs themselves. Some abbreviations may be read in various ways if not made clear by the context; for example, "chlor.," which may be read "chloralum," "chloridum" or "chloras"; "sulf.," which may be read "sulfur," "sulfidum" or "sulfas'; and "ext. col.," which may be read "extractum colchici" or "extractum colocynthidis."

Most publications are now aiding the campaign in behalf of metric measurements and urge their use in prescriptions. Metric measurements alone are used whenever possible, or the metric values are given first, followed by the apothecaries' equivalents. If the apothecaries' units must for any reason be given first, metric equivalents are always inserted after them. It is particularly bad form to mix two systems of measurements, as: "Dissolve 10 gm of

―――― in 2 fluidounces of water," or "100 cc contains 30 grains of ――――." (In certain areas such as pharmacy, "milliliters" is now often preferred to "cubic centimeters.")

To avoid confusion, grams is abbreviated gm; grains is written in full except when lack of space necessitates abbreviation, in which case "gr.," with a lower case "g," is used.

11
BIBLIOGRAPHIC MATERIAL

THE MEASURE of a medical publication's vitality has been said to be the frequency with which it is referred to by later publications. In 1960, one authority compared the age of all references included in two journals of biology over a ten-year period. In one periodical, less than half of the references cited dated farther back than five years. Another study of the obsolescence of scientific articles covering a number of periodicals found a half-life of approximately four to 12 years for references. Writer D. J. DeSola Price has said that a scientific manuscript can be considered obsolete ten years after publication.

Many attempts have been made to determine the significance and importance of individual medical periodicals by counting the number of references made to a given periodical in a given year. In a review of this subject, Dr. Renata Tagliacozzo of the University of Michigan remarks that the number of papers published by a scientist or group of scientists is often used to evaluate the performance of either the scientists or their institution. But mere quantity is an unreliable indication. An Einstein work on relativity is not to be balanced against 100 papers by an unknown who has multiplied one unimportant observation into many published reports.

The significance with which a scientific paper is cited by other independent writers—a citation count—is a better measure of the importance of a piece of research than simply a rough count of a total number of publications. If a field of science is growing rapidly, stimulated by original discoveries, its importance is promptly reflected by citations in bibliographies. Dr. Tagliacozzo calls attention to the *Science Citation Index,* produced by the Institute for Scientific Information in Philadelphia, which draws material from over 1,500 periodicals, both American and foreign, and is said to include all the items published in each journal except advertising and news. This index has been published quarterly with an annual cumulation since 1964. The size of the index for 1966 is estimated at three million citations. Similar indexes have been developed for statistics, mathematics and various aspects of chemistry and physics.

A number of studies in the dissemination of technical information using computers are being made under the auspices of various universities. A study of the *Science Citation Index* is cited by Dr. Tagliacozzo to determine how "noisy" a citation network may be. The jargon word "noisy" relates to the irrelevant information retrieved along with relevant information in a *Science Citation Index*. The study found that two out of seven retrieved articles were relevant and the other five were not.

But questions still remain. What differentiates citations which die a natural death from citations which die a premature death? How can citations that disappear because of lack of vitality be separated from those included in or replaced by later work?

A periodical with a captive circulation may have fewer readers and thereby fewer citations than a subscription periodical with a small circulation. A periodical distributed gratis may show a large circulation and a large readership and yet fail to be measurable in significance by a citation count. A periodical devoted to publishing new observations rapidly may not be cited as often as one devoted to publishing long contributions full of data, with records of experiments and many tables.

With the mechanization of storage and retrieval still undergoing experimentation and study, the time is too soon to evaluate citation indexes. Their evaluation will continue to be difficult until their capacities and limitations are known by actual trial and until the best ways of utilizing them and the types of users to whom they are best suited are determined.

SECURING A BIBLIOGRAPHY

In investigating the literature on a subject, begin preferably with the most accessible indexes. *The Journal of the American*

Medical Association publishes at the end of each volume an index of the original articles appearing in its pages and of articles in other periodicals that have been abstracted in *The Journal* during the previous six months. Many of the articles there mentioned will contain references to other articles, these in turn mentioning still others. Thus, more and more references are accumulated, until perhaps one finds an article by a reliable writer who has summarized the literature to the date of his publication.

The Quarterly Cumulative Index Medicus

If a more complete study of a subject is contemplated, the *Quarterly Cumulative Index Medicus,* formerly published by the American Medical Association, should be consulted. This is a consolidation of the *Index Medicus,* established in 1879 by J. S. Billings and Robert Fletcher, and the *Quarterly Cumulative Index,* launched in 1916 by the American Medical Association. In 1927 the two publications merged under the title *Quarterly Cumulative Index Medicus.* From 1927 to 1931, inclusive, the index was published jointly by the American Medical Association and the Army Medical Library. After 1932 it was supported and published entirely by the American Medical Association. In it, all authors are listed alphabetically, with sufficient cross-indexing to make the finding of references simple.

This index was at first published four times a year, the first and third numbers being temporary (bound in paper) and each covering periodicals received during a three-month period; the second and fourth numbers (bound in cloth) covered periodicals received during a half-year. Each number was published as soon as possible after the completion of the period covered; but publication was suspended temporarily with the Jan.-June 1954 volume. With the establishment of the National Medical Library, its computerized index *Medlars,* became the chief reference source.

The Current List of Medical Literature

The original *Current List of Medical Literature* was founded in 1941 by Dr. Atherton Seidell as a venture of the Friends of the Army Medical Library. In 1945 the *Current List of Medical Lit-*

erature became an official government publication of the Army Medical Library. In July, 1950, the first issue of the completely refurbished monthly *Current List of Medical Literature* appeared. Many changes have been made in the intervening years; however, the dual arrangement consisting of a Register of Articles and a separate index referring to the Register has remained the same.

The Index-Catalogue of the Library of the Surgeon General's Office

The Armed Forces Medical Library, formerly the Library of the Surgeon General's Office, contains the greatest collection of medical periodicals, pamphlets and books in any medical library in America. In 1876 John Shaw Billings published a specimen sheet of a combined index-catalogue, with authors and subjects arranged in alphabetical order. Established by act of the Congress of the United States in 1879, the first volume of the *Index-Catalogue of the Library of the Surgeon General's Office* was issued in 1880. This work has now been discontinued, but in 1955 it had reached its fifty-third volume and its fourth alphabetical set, covering the entire material in the Armed Forces Medical Library as of 1955. There is in the library an index on file cards which is kept up to date.

In 1956 Congress passed a bill transferring the Armed Forces Medical Library to the National Library of Medicine.

HOW TO SECURE THE COMPLETE LITERATURE

If the complete literature on a subject is desired, one will do well to begin with the available volumes of the *Index-Catalogue of the Library of the Surgeon General's Office*. Having secured the references listed therein, one may then consult the volumes of the *Index Medicus* and the *Quarterly Cumulative Index* as far as they go, and the index to the bound volumes of the *Journal of the American Medical Association* up to 1916. The references may then be brought up to recent date with the aid of the *Quarterly Cumulative Index Medicus* and the *Current Medical List* followed by *Medlars* and the indexes of *Excerpta Medica*.

It is seldom desirable to review the complete literature on a subject in an article for publication in a periodical. The science of medicine has grown so vastly and its book and periodical literature is so extensive that complete reviews repeat themselves endlessly in the literature.

It is no longer excusable to bolster a report of a case or an article with a compilation of references to all similar cases that have been reported in the literature. The growth of medical literature has made this not only a useless but also an unwarranted task. Reference should be given only to articles that illuminate the subject. Hardly any one detail of a well-prepared and well-written article will give a better and clearer idea of a writer's methods or foster greater confidence in the accuracy and soundness of his views than well-chosen, well-arranged, absolutely correct references. References should be given only to articles that have been directly utilized by the author presenting them. To republish long bibliographies taken from other authors is a form of plagiarism which unnecessarily burdens the literature.

SECURING MEDICAL PERIODICALS

A physician who has access to a good medical library probably will be able to find bound volumes of the most important medical periodicals. If he wants to consult the more recent literature, he may order periodicals published in the United States directly from the publishers. On making proper deposit, a physician may arrange to borrow publications from the National Library of Medicine.

ARRANGEMENT AND FORM OF BIBLIOGRAPHIC REFERENCES

Footnotes

Footnotes which refer to the article as a whole are placed on the title page. An asterisk or a dagger is used only when it is necessary definitely to connect the footnote with one author or with a specific part of the title. Ordinarily, an asterisk is used for the first footnote that requires a special designation and a dagger for the second. A dagger is always used, however, for a footnote recording the death of an author. Such a footnote should read: "Dr Brown died on March 10, 1948." When a paper has been read at a meeting of a society, a footnote to that effect should be given.

VITAMIN C AND PIGMENT
THEODORE BROOKS, M.D.

From the Department of Dermatology, College of Medicine, University of Illinois, service of Dr. F. E. Sampson.

Read before the Section on Dermatology and Syphilology at the Eighty-Seventh Annual Session of the American Medical Association, Kansas City, Mo., May 14, 1936.

ANATOMIC FEATURES OF THE CARDIAC ORIFICE OF THE STOMACH
WITH SPECIAL REFERENCE TO CARDIOSPASM
FREDERICK C. LENDRUM, M.D., PH.D.*

Abridgment of a thesis submitted to the faculty of the Graduate School of the University of Minnesota in partial fulfilment of the requirements for the degree of Doctor of Philosophy in Medicine.

PATHOGENESIS OF NONCASEATING TUBERCULOSIS OF THE SKIN AND LYMPH NODES
RALPH R. MELLON, M.D.
and
LAWRENCE G. BEINHAUER, M.D.

From the Institute of Pathology (Dr. Mellon) and the Department of Dermatology (Dr. Beinhauer) of the Western Pennsylvania Hospital.

An author's affiliation may be included after his name on the title page, as in the following examples:

LAUREN V. ACKERMAN, M.D.
Assitant Professor of Pathology
Washington University School of Medicine
St. Louis, Missouri

MORRIS MOORE, M.D.
Mycologist to the Barnard Free Skin and Cancer Hospital
St. Louis, Missouri

---

*Former Fellow in Medicine, the Mayo Foundation.

References to the literature and comments on various matters mentioned in an article that are to be used as footnotes should be numbered consecutively throughout the article, with corresponding superior reference figures in the text. When the same reference is used twice, instead of duplicating the note or using the words "loc. cit.," it is better to repeat in the text the number of the original note. When an author wishes to refer to several articles at one point, he should combine them in one footnote or mention the authors' names individually in the text, with one superior figure for each. If several references combined in one footnote are referred to individually later, they may be numbered *a, b.* etc.

When necessary to eliminate a footnote after the type is set, the numbers of succeeding footnotes should be changed if there are not too many involved. However, if there would need to be a great number of changes, the superior figure—say 6—in the text should be deleted, so that the reader will not look to the foot of the page needlessly, and "6. Footnote deleted on proof" should be substituted for the discarded reference. Conversely, if an author finds it necessary to insert a footnote after the type is set—say between 10 and 11—the reference may be numbered "10a" so that the numbers of the following footnotes need not be changed.

A note appended to an article after the type is set, unless it is a mere footnote, is considered to be a part of the text matter and is set in body type. If it contains bibliographic references, they should be treated as footnotes, numbered consecutively following the last footnote in the text.

Since in the printed article footnotes appear at the bottom of the page on which they are mentioned in the text, in the preparation of the manuscript they should be typed, in double space, at the bottom of the page on which they are cited.

Bibliographies

References are grouped at the end of a paper in the form of a bibliography only when an exhaustive review of the literature has been made on a subject of sufficient importance to warrant such a survey. The references constituting a bibliography may be arranged either alphabetically or chronologically, or in exceptional instances according to some other logical scheme. The alphabetical arrangement is usually preferable, for it makes it easy for the reader to locate an author's name quickly.

Other References

References in Society Proceedings, Discussions and Legends for Illustrations

Footnotes are not used in discussions of original articles or in society proceedings. References should be incorporated in the text, in parentheses. The form used is the same as that for references used as footnotes except that the names of periodicals are italicized.

When a reference mentioned in a legend is cited in the text also, the superior figure designating the footnote to the text may be used in the legend instead of repeating the reference (example A, following). When a reference given in a legend is not cited in the text, it should be incorporated in the legend (examples B and C, following). (It cannot safely be numbered consecutively with the footnotes in the text because until the printed pages are made up it is difficult to determine where an illustration will be inserted.) When one reference is mentioned in several legends but not in the text, it may be possible to include a sentence concerning it in the text and to insert a footnote; a superior figure may then be used each time the reference is cited.

The following examples of legends are in the proper form:

> A. Figure 1. *A* is a demonstration of suture method 4, the Halsted presection suture technic, used only on the anterior aspect of the ostium. *B* is a demonstration of suture method 5, the ordinary continuous circular through and through suture, which when used anteriorly inevitably causes macroscopic mucosal eversion, as shown at *a* (Martzloff and Suckow[1]).
>
> B. Figure 10. In the middle of the figure is a myelophage *(M)*, which is a large vacuolated body, the processes *(P)* of which emanate from the nucleus *(N)*, an oligodendrocyte forming a ring around the enclosures of myelin (two dark fragments). This section (Hassin, George B.: Histopathologic findings in a case of superior and inferior polioencephalitis. *Arch. Neurol. Psychiat.,* 5:552, May, 1921) is from

the brain of a patient with so-called superior and inferior polioencephalitis. Bielschowsky's stain; × 1,200.

C. Figure 1. *A, B* and *C,* dorsal views of brains of rabbits showing areas of cortex removed in three experiments. *D,* dorsal view of the brain of a rabbit, in which the area outlined by a broken line represents the precentral motor area as shown by C. Winkler and A. Potter *(An Anatomical Guide to Experimental Researches on the Rabbit's Brain.* Amsterdam, W. Versluys, 1911). The numbers on the opposite hemisphere indicate points stimulated to obtain movements of (1) the face and jaws, (2) the head and neck and (3) the scapula.

When material is reproduced from another source, permission for reproduction should be secured from the author and the publisher, for the better periodicals and books are copyrighted.

References in Tables

Frequently bibliographic references for authors are listed in a table. Such references cannot be assigned numbers consecutive with those in the text, as it is impossible to tell where a table will be inserted on the printed page. This plan may result in a slight inconsistency of form. The alternative, however—that of including all the references in the table when only some of them are cited in the text—has the disadvantage of failing to indicate to the reader that certain references are mentioned in the text as well as in the table and of making the table occupy more space.

TABLE 3
Normal Range of Venous Pressure in Adults

Observer	Method	Range, Mm Water
Owens, L. B.: *J. Lab Clin. Med., 18:*266, 1932	Indirect	35–90
Eyster, J. E. A., and Middleton, W. S.: *Arch. Int. Med., 34:*228, Aug., 1924	Indirect	50–60
Runge, H.: *Arch. f. Gynäk., 22:*142, 1924	Indirect	48–66
Moritz and von Tabora[4]	Direct	40–80
Berghausen, O.: *J. Med., 15:*22, 1934	Direct	40–80
Caughey[5b]	Direct	40–80

References to periodicals in tables should include the name of the author, his initials, the name of the periodical and the volume, page and year. The title should not be included unless there is special reason. References to books should be in the usual complete form.

The method of inserting footnotes other than bibliographic references in tables will be discussed in Chapter 14.

Form for References

An incorrect reference may cause the reader to waste much time in looking for an article. It leads, moreover, to the assumption that the author did not actually consult the work but copied the reference. The author should ensure accuracy by seeing each article himself and verifying the data. Special attention should be given to the spelling of foreign names and of words in foreign titles. Accents should be included as they appear in the names and titles cited. An English title should be quoted exactly unless there is an error that is obviously typographic. The accuracy of a reference is further substantiated by making it complete.

A complete reference to a book contains the following information (example 5 in the list—see page 127):

1. Author's surname and initials.
2. Title of the book (capitalize all main words).
3. Edition.
4. Place of publication.
5. Name of the publisher.
6. Year of publication.
7. Volume, if more than one has been published.
8. Page.

A complete reference to an article in a periodical contains:

1. Author's surname and initials.
2. Title of the article (capitalize only initial word and proper nouns in English).
3. Name of the periodical, abbreviated according to the form given in the *Quarterly Cumulative Index Medicus* or written correctly in full (an abbreviation devised by an individual author is likely to lead to confusion).
4. Volume.
5. Page.
6. Month—and day of the month if the periodical is published more often than once a month.
7. Year.

The year and the volume number may serve as a check on each other. The page number permits quick reference when the volume is at hand. The date is important, especially if the reference is to a recent periodical, which is likely not to be bound. It is useful also if one desires to purchase a number of the periodical, for a publisher prefers to have the exact date of issue rather than the volume and the page. Some periodicals—for instance, the *British Medical Journal* and the *Lancet*—do not use volume numbers except 1 and 2 for each year.

In references to bulletins published by the various departments of the United States government, the following information should be included, in this order:

1. Name of the author.
2. Title of the bulletin.
3. Number of the bulletin.
4. Name of the department.
5. Name of the bureau.
6. Date.

References to these and to other bulletins, monographs and reports should be treated as are references to books, without undue use of abbreviations. The exact title should always be given, and the serial number, the name of the series of bulletins or monographs (written correctly in full), the publisher and the date should be included.

A few general principles in regard to form may be mentioned:[1]

1. Titles of articles and of books are not abbreviated.
2. If possible titles should be given in the language in which they originally appeared. If for some reason an author wishes to translate the title into English, however, the translations should be accurate and all the foreign titles should be translated.
3. Italics are not used to distinguish titles of books, articles or periodicals in footnotes, legends or bibliographies.
4. The names of all the authors should be given unless there are more than four or unless the names cannot be obtained.

---

[1] The methods indicated are those followed by the periodicals published by the American Medical Association. Other periodicals have individual styles, which vary somewhat from those listed. A contributor should acquaint himself with the form used by the periodical to which his paper is to be submitted.

5. The number of a periodical usually is not included when the volume number is available.
6. Foreign words of reference, such as *tome* (volume), *fascicolo* (part), *Seite* (page), *Teil* (part), *Auflage* (edition), *Abteilung* (section or part), *Band* (volume), *Heft* (number), *Beiheft* (supplement) and *Lieferung* (part or number), should be translated.
7. References to abstracts of articles should be included only (1) when the author wishes to show that he has consulted an abstract rather than the original article or (2) when the original article appeared in a journal that is not readily accessible to the majority of physicians. In these instances complete data for the original article should be included as well as the reference for the abstract.
8. It usually is sufficient to give the number of the first page of the material cited. If, however, an author wishes to give both the first and the last page, he should use this form for all the references in his article. Occasionally an author wants to give not the page on which the article begins but the specific page on which the material cited appears. If the policy is followed, a note to that effect should be included, for the reader normally expects the page cited to be the first one of the article.

12
PREPARATION OF THE MANUSCRIPT

THE GENERAL APPEARANCE of a manuscript has a psychologic effect on an editor. A manuscript carelessly arranged, without pagination, composed of sheets of various sizes, with additions written on slips pinned or clipped to the pages or with corrections made without regard to neatness or to clarity may prejudice the reader who is to pass on its merits. Slovenly preparation has caused the return of numerous manuscripts which otherwise might have been accepted.

Authors may well devote some time to learning the rudiments of printing. Such knowledge helps in the preparation of the manuscript and saves many needless corrections. Authors, however, are not expected to specify the type to be used, any more than patients are expected to specify the diagnostic tests to be undertaken.

Paper

The paper used should be of standard size ($8\frac{1}{2}$ by 11 inches), nontransparent and of good quality, so that it will withstand handling.

Original and Carbon Copies

The original copy of a paper should be submitted if at all possible. If not, a first carbon copy on good paper may be acceptable. Editors need good, clean copy for practical reasons. Each manuscript is read by at least one editor and then, in turn, by the copy editor, the typesetter and the proofreader or the copyholder. With the exception of the editor, each of these must check spelling, punctuation, capitalization and grammatical construction.

Some publications ask for both the original and a carbon copy. The latter is used for corrections and queries to the author; final changes are correlated in the editorial office and then indicated on the original, with typographic instructions, so that the typesetter can work from a clear copy.

The wise author will always retain a carbon copy, both for safety and to compare with the proof. This will show him what changes have been made and perhaps indicate faults in his writing. In this manner he may indirectly secure helpful criticism.

Typing the Manuscript

A manuscript should never be typed single spaced. No matter how well the paper is written or how carefully it is prepared, the keen eye of the copy editor may find typographic errors, misspelled words, or grammatical slips that require interlineation. This is done with difficulty on closely typed manuscripts (see Fig. 1.) Typing should therefore be double- or even triple-spaced, the latter being preferred by some publications.

Liberal margins should be left on all sides—at least $1\frac{1}{2}$ inches at top and left and 1 inch at bottom and right. The author should use the margins to indicate the placement of illustrations, tables, charts, etc.

Neatness

Illegibility, smudging or other marked defects in the preparation of a manuscript may give the impression that the research or observation described in the article was equally slipshod and inaccurate and may turn the scale against its acceptance.

A manuscript should be folded, not rolled. When it consists of too many sheets to permit of easy folding, it should be sent flat.

Author's Name

The name and address of the author should appear on each page of the manuscript and on each illustration, chart and table. The title of the article, the author's name and degrees, his appointments, and his address should be typed on one page. This information should follow as closely as possible the style of articles in the publication to which the manuscript is to be sent. The various items should be separated by sufficient space to permit indication of type sizes and corrections. A 3-inch (7.5 cm) margin at the upper edge of the first page should be allowed, as printing instructions are written there by manuscript editors. An example follows:

A REVIEW OF FOUR HUNDRED AND FORTY CASES OF PELLAGRA
V. P. SYDENSTRICKER, M.D.
AND
E. S. ARMSTRONG, M.D.

From the University of Georgia School of Medicine and the University Hospital, Augusta, Georgia.

The author's office or residence address (street and number) may be placed at the end of his article if he wishes to include it.

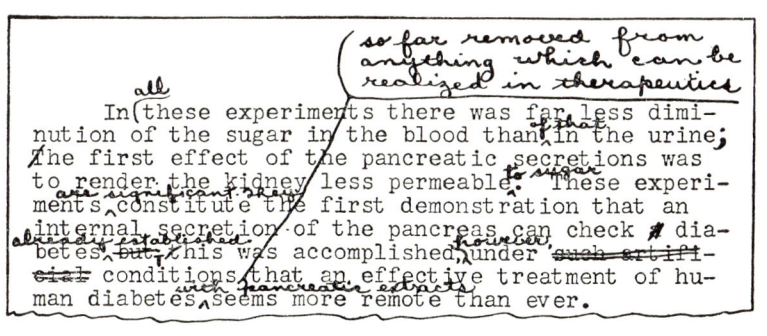

Figure 1. Several of the worst mechanical corrections are illustrated here: single spacing, insufficient margins and corrections that are crowded and hard to read.

General Rules

In summary, the following directions for preparing a manuscript are important:
1. Use unglazed white paper of good quality, $8\frac{1}{2}$ by 11 inches in size.
2. Type in double or triple space on only one side of the paper, leaving good margins on all sides.

                    all:
        In ~~these~~ experiments there was far

    less diminution of the sugar in the blood
            of that
    than ~~in~~ the urine; ~~T~~he first effect of

    the pancreatic secretions was to render
                            to sugar.
    the kidney less permeable. These experi-
            are significant. They
    ments ~~constitute~~ the first demonstration

    that an internal secretion of the pan-
                        already established.
    creas can check ~~a~~ diabetes ~~but~~ this was
            however,
    accomplished, under ~~such artificial~~ con-
    so far removed from anything which can be realized in
    ditions ~~that~~ an effective treatment of   *therapeu-*
                    with pancreatic extracts   *tics*
    human diabetes seems more remote than ever.

Figure 2. Wide spacing and ample margins give opportunity for legible corrections.

produced   *or*
                                                    almost
        The diabetes in animals by complete
complete,
    ~~removal~~ of the pancreas so closely re-

    sembles human diabetes in ~~all~~ its essential

    features that it seems reasonable to hope

        that any method~~s~~ which will cure the for-
    of use   *against*
        mer will ~~also~~ be ~~useful in~~ the latter. ;
l.c. Any light which may be obtained on the

        experimental form~~s~~ will ~~also~~ help to a

    better understanding of the human disease.

Figure 3. This manuscript has been corrected as if it were proof, using guide lines which make it unnecessarily hard to read. Figure 4 shows proper way to make corrections in manuscript.

> produced   or almost
> The diabetes ^in animals by complete)
> complete,
> (removal of the pancreas so closely re-
> sembles human diabetes in ~~all~~ its essential
> features that it seems reasonable to hope
> that any method$ which will cure the for-
>   of use against
> mer will ~~also~~ be (~~useful in~~ the latter;
> /Any light which may be obtained on the
> experimental form$ will ~~also~~ help to a
> better understanding of the human disease.

Figure 4. This manuscript has been corrected properly.

3. Type tables on separate sheets, as these usually are set on a different typesetting machine from the text. Indicate in the margin of the text where each table should be inserted.
4. Type footnotes (also double-spaced) on separate sheets at the end of the article or chapter or immediately after their text references, depending on the practice of the periodical to which the article is submitted. Be sure they agree in number with their respective references in the text.
5. Type legends for illustrations on a separate sheet at the end of the manuscript. Number the legends in sequence to agree with the illustrations.
6. Type quoted material double spaced, using quotation marks for short excerpts. Quotations more than a few lines long should begin on a new line, and their exact extent should be indicated by a vertical line in the left margin. Obtain written permission from the copyright holder.
7. Number sheets in consecutive order in the upper right hand corner.
8. Fasten sheets together with pins, clips or other easily removable fasteners. Do not submit manuscripts that have

been permanently bound, as this makes for difficult handling by editors, compositors and proofreaders.
9. Do not paste, pin or clip illustrations to manuscript. Do not write heavily on the backs of photographs so that the impression will show on the reverse side. If necessary for identification, write lightly in the margin.
10. Number the illustrations in sequence and indicate in the margin of the text where they are to be inserted.
11. Indicate paragraphs clearly, either by the usual indention or by the use of the paragraph mark, ¶.
12. Make all corrections on manuscript in pencil.
13. Put any necessary corrections between the typewritten lines of the manuscript, using a caret to indicate place of insertion. Retype any sheet bearing numerous corrections.
14. Draw a horizontal line through words or phrases to be deleted. If several paragraphs or pages are to be eliminated, draw an oblique line through such matter.
15. If several pages are deleted from the manuscript, the pages should be either renumbered or so numbered at the top as to indicate the omission. For example, if three pages are deleted (pages 25 to 27), the page following 24 may be marked "25-28." If a page is inserted—say between pages 5 and 6—it may be marked "5a" with the notation "Page 5a follows" at the bottom of page 5 and "Page 5a precedes" at the top of page 6.
16. Mark off by brackets any material to be transposed from one portion of the manuscript to another, indicating the transposition by the notation "Transpose to page —." On the latter page, clearly indicate where the transposed material is to be inserted, with the notation "Insert from page —." Better yet, cut the copy apart and paste in the inserts where they belong or retype the material in correct order, as printers find this easier to handle.
17. Write the word "End" at the bottom of the last page of the manuscript. Also state at this point whether or not there will be an index.
18. Submit the original typing to the publisher, retaining a carbon copy for comparative reading.

13
ILLUSTRATIONS

Good pictures are eloquent; frequently one small illustration will convey more to the reader than could be explained in several pages of text matter. Such an illustration nearly always has evolved from a thorough understanding of the material and a well-chosen attitude from which to present it. Many authors, however, submit huge numbers of illustrations with their manuscripts, regardless of whether or not the pictures are necessary to bring out adequately the points made in the text and even regardless of whether they bring out any point at all. Few journals can afford to reproduce large numbers of illustrations. Therefore, unless the author is willing to contribute toward the costs of reproduction of his illustrations, he should curtail the use of pictures as much as possible, selecting for reproduction only those which he feels are required to illustrate points to be emphasized. Care in planning illustrations will reduce their number materially, and the omission of extensive backgrounds will reduce the size of the finished engraving, which governs its cost.

Readers of scientific journals may be assumed to be familiar with the normal appearances, gross and microscopic, of the various organs; hence illustrations of normal conditions should be used only when required for the sake of contrast. The first rule regarding illustrations, therefore, is that they should *illustrate*. Only after this function has been fulfilled may the artistic elements be considered.

PREPARATION OF ILLUSTRATIONS

In preparing illustrations for publication, the author should consider the size of the type column and the size of the page of the periodical in which the article may appear. The illustrations should be of a size that, with reasonable reduction, can be accommodated to the type column.

Sometimes pictures can be grouped to advantage, thus permitting saving of space and expense. For instance, three blocks $2\frac{1}{4}$ inches (6.3 cm) wide by 3 inches (7.5 cm) high will cost more than one block in which the same three illustrations are combined. Two of the pictures could be placed side by side, making a cut less than 5 inches (12.5 cm) wide and the third block centered above or below. A better appearance is secured if single pictures or groups of pictures are higher than they are wide, as is the page of most periodicals.

Illustrations should be suitably numbered and their position in the manuscript should be indicated even though it is not always possible for the printer to follow these directions implicitly. The number of the picture and the name of the author should appear on each, and the top should be marked. Labels for identification of illustrations may be procured from stationers. These should be large enough to provide space on which may be recorded the names of both the author and the journal in which the article is intended to appear, the number of the figure and any instructions concerning reduction or reproduction that it is deemed desirable to furnish. It is inadvisable to write on the back of a photograph, since this may mar its surface. If, however, labels are not available and it is necessary to write on the back for purposes of identification, a soft pencil should be used and little pressure applied.

Since medical illustration in recent years has attained such a high standard of perfection, any article illustrated by amateurish pictures suffers by comparison with the other articles in almost any journal. This is also true of photography. Competent medical illustrators are available in nearly every large city today; if not, artists can be recommended by the editors or publishers. Early consultation between author and artist will result in useful illustrations.

When the illustrations constitute a major part of a paper, their suitability to a simple type of reproduction may be a factor in the acceptance or rejection of the manuscript. Here the experienced artist, familiar with photoengraving methods, can render substantial aid to both author and publisher.

The artist should be given all available information concerning the journal in which the article is planned to appear. Page size, column width, etc., are important in planning the drawing size and the amount of reduction necessary.

Photographs and drawings intended for periodicals are preferably mounted with rubber cement on white cardboard, leaving margins all around on which technical directions may be added. If the mounts are uniform, packaging is simplified. Book publishers often prefer to mount illustrations themselves according to the makeup planned.

Clips or pins should not be used to fasten photographs, particularly glossy prints. They leave impressions or holes in the photographs which cannot be eradicated in reproduction.

Illustrations should be sent flat—never rolled or folded—and protected with cardboard. A crease made in folding cannot be eradicated in the process of reproduction and will mar the surface of the picture.

LABELING ILLUSTRATIONS

After the illustration has been prepared, the author should make certain that the significant points are clearly apparent and that they will come to the attention of the reader. Special attention can be called to these points either by a special reference in the legend to appear under the picture or by lettering placed on the photograph itself.

Letters, words and numbers placed on the surface of the picture should be sufficiently large to be legible when reduced to the size indicated and should be neatly made, with a view to securing a pleasing appearance after reproduction; hence a plain, open-faced style is preferred.

Judicious use of labels incorporated in the drawing and fully spelled out should not detract from the appearance of the drawing. The use of coded labels (*a, b, c,* etc., or *1, 2, 3,* etc.) with their interpretation in the legend under the illustration is apt to dis-

152 Medical Writing

courage the careful study of the picture by causing the eyes to be constantly shifted. (Compare Figs. 5A and 5B).

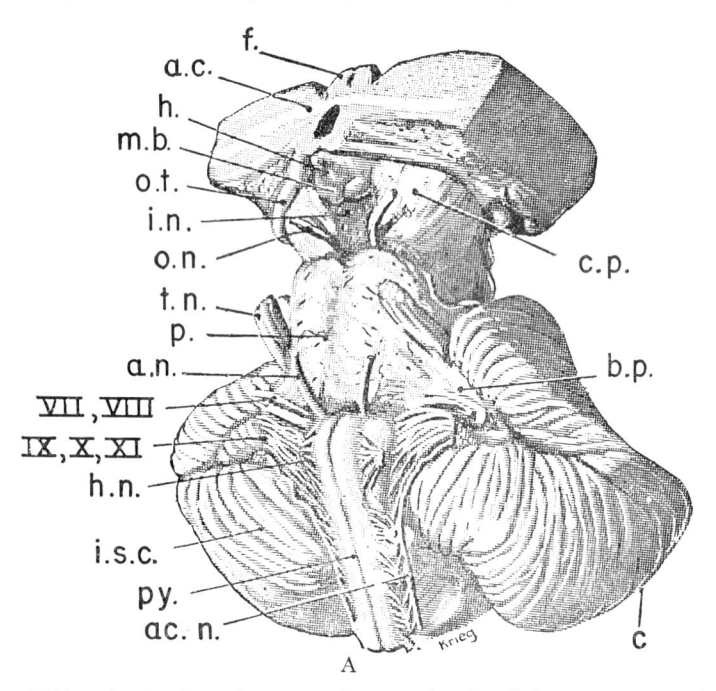

Figure 5(A). (a.c.) Anterior commissure, (a.n.) abducent nerve, (ac.n.) accessory nerve, (b.p.) brachium pontus, (c.) cerebellum, (c.p.) cerebral peduncle, (f.) fornix, (h.) hypothalamus, (h.n.) hypoglossal nerve, (i.n.) interpeduncular nucleus, (i.s.c.) inferior surface of cerebellum, (m.b.) mamillary bodies, (o.n.) oculomotor nerve, (o.t.) optic tract, (p.) pons, (py.) pyramid, (t.n.) trigeminal nerve; (VII, VIII, IX, X, XI) 7th, 8th, 9th, 10th, 11th cranial nerves. (Use of abbreviated labels forces reader to shift from figure to legend for interpretation.) Compare this with Figure 5 (B). (Kreig: *Functional Neuroanatomy*. New York, Blackiston Division, McGraw-Hill [with modified side labels]).

Labels should be placed so as to require as little extra space as possible, and thus not increase the cost of reproduction. It is generally desirable, therefore, to place black letters on unessential white areas within the picture or white letters on black areas, making the dotted lines and the lettering come entirely within the body of the photograph.

Illustrations

[Figure: labeled anatomical illustration B with labels: Fornix, Ante. commissure, Hypothalamus, Mammillary bodies, Optic tract, Interpeduncular nuc., Oculomotor nerve, Trigeminal nerve, Pons, Abducent nerve, VII, VIII nerves, IX, X, XI nerves, Hypoglossal nerve, Inferior surface of cerebellum, Pyramid, Accessory nerve, Cerebral peduncle, Brachium pontis, Cerebellum]

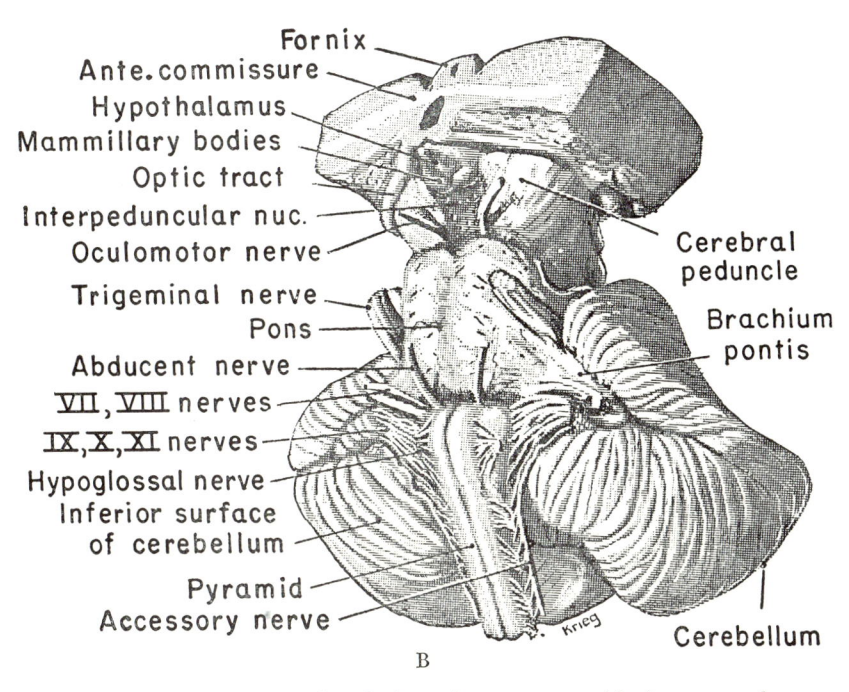

Figure 5 (B). Here the reader finds each structure with its name close at hand. The vertical column space occupied by this figure is the same as Figure 5 (A), and the space taken up by the legend below Figure 5 (A) has been saved here. (Kreig: *Functional Neuroanatomy*. New York, Blakiston Division, McGraw-Hill.)

When abbreviations in labels are necessary, only standard abbreviations should be used (m., a., v., n., for muscle, artery, vein, nerve, respectively; and inf., sup., int., ext., in anatomic terms are acceptable). Consistency in the use of some standard terminology will add to the value of a series of illustrations, especially since these same illustrations may later be borrowed by other authors.

The lettering may be done by a competent draftsman, or printed characters may be obtained to be pasted on the illustrations. These characters, however, while usually satisfactory from the point of view of appearance, do not always adhere to the illustration—particularly to a glossy surface. Sometimes they are lost after the pictures pass through the editorial office, and the loss is not detected until the author receives the proof. Any insertions or changes after the blocks have been made require the making of a new block and mean added expense.

Perhaps the best method of marking points to be indicated by guide lines and side labels is to cover the illustration or photograph with a sheet of tracing paper, transparent enough to be easily seen through, on which the author may mark his choice of those structures to which the reader's attention is to be called. This permits the editor to use either the side or the top or bottom margin for the lettering necessary to identify the structures. If guide lines have already been ruled on the illustration by the author, it frequently happens that not enough space has been left for the lettering which is to appear at the end of each line.

LEGENDS

A full descriptive legend to be placed beneath each picture should be provided. The legends should be numbered in sequence to correspond with the pictures and should be typewritten on a separate sheet at the end of the manuscript, not on the illustrations. They must be given the same care in composition and in expression as is the material in the body of the article. The legend should explain fully all the important points brought out by the illustration and identify each of the letters, numbers, arrows or other marks included within the picture.

PERMISSIONS

Many people object to having their photographs published in scientific periodicals. The author of an article containing such a photograph either should secure from the patient written permission for publication and inform the editor of the periodical to which the article is submitted that written permission has been secured, or should mask the face in the portrait by blocking out the eyes with India ink or by pasting over them pieces of paper of a neutral color. If pictures depicting conditions about the eyes accompany a paper, the patient's written consent to the use of his or her photograph must be secured since the picture would be useless were the eyes blocked out.

When photographs are submitted as scientific proof, photographers must be informed that retouching is not to be done on them. However, careful retouching by a competent artist will often clarify the contents of other photographs whose details are visible to one familiar with the case, yet too vague to be useful to the reader.

Frequently an author wishes to use one or more illustrations that have been published elsewhere. In such instances the author should secure written permission from the original author or from the publisher, since the better periodicals and books are copyrighted. A statement that written permission has been obtained should accompany the manuscript when it is submitted for publication. Otherwise the publisher will be put to the trouble of asking the author if such permission has been granted, and this usually causes delay in publication. Complete information (see chapter entitled "Bibliographic Material" for definition of a complete reference) concerning the source of the illustrations should be included either in the legend or in a footnote. The author should be sure that borrowed illustrations do not contain contradictions to statements made in his paper.

CHOICE OF MEDIUM FOR REPRODUCTION

Line drawings made with pen and ink on bristol board or black lithograph pencil on rough or stipple paper can be reproduced as zinc line engravings, which cost from a half to a third as much as halftones (see Fig. 6). Drawings of this sort must be made with pure black ink, or in the case of lithograph pencil, the strokes must be placed firmly so as to produce pure black patterns. Shading on such drawings must be made by lines, cross hatching or stippling, or by the use of Ben Day tints or shading film (see page 156.)

Photographs or drawings that have been prepared properly lend themselves to satisfactory reproduction by the halftone process. This method must be used if lines of tones intermediate between black and white are used in drawing. (See pages 157-158.)

Zinc Line Engravings

Zinc line engravings are used in the reproduction of line drawings (See figure 6) and of printed matter appearing in black

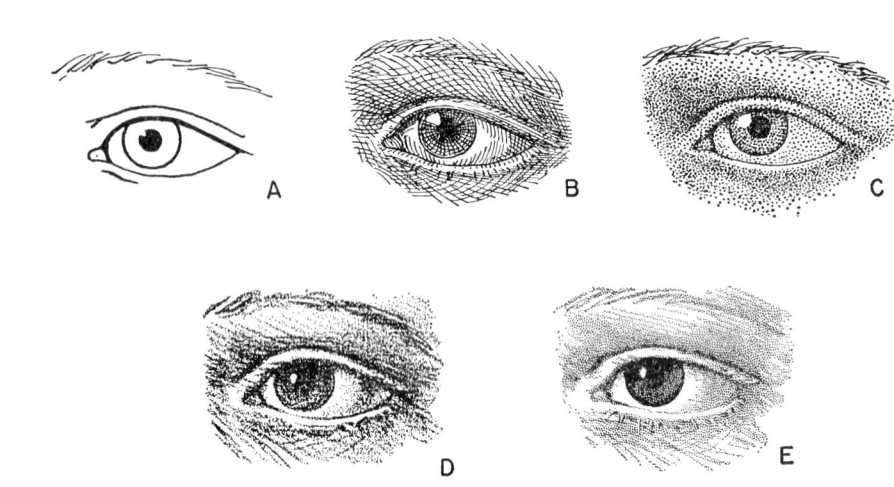

Figure 6. Various art techniques suitable for reproduction by the zinc line engraving process. (A) Simple outline of structures. (B) Lines and crosshatching for differentiation of parts. (C) Stippling to explain form by light and shade. (D) Lithograph pencil on rough paper, with corneal reflex painted in with Chinese white. (E) Lithograph pencil on no. 1 Ross Stipple Board. In this drawing the iris of the eye was painted solid black, and by lightly scratching the tops of the stipples, a much darker tone was produced than could be secured with pencil alone. The corneal reflex has been scratched out.

and white. The original drawing is preferred to a photograph of it, since some of the clearness and detail are lost each time an illustration is submitted to a photographic process.

Drawings made with ordinary lead pencil are rarely reproduced satisfactorily by this method; as a rule they must be returned for redrawing or be reproduced by the halftone process.

The process of reducing will soften the drawing and give the reproduction a more finished appearance. Drawings should be neatly done; straight lines should be made with a ruler and circles with a compass. The average physician, not having had the training of a draftsman, usually is not competent to make creditable drawings. Therefore, most medical periodicals cooperate with the author by having a competent artist do the work for him from a rough sketch that may be submitted (see Figs. 7 and 8).

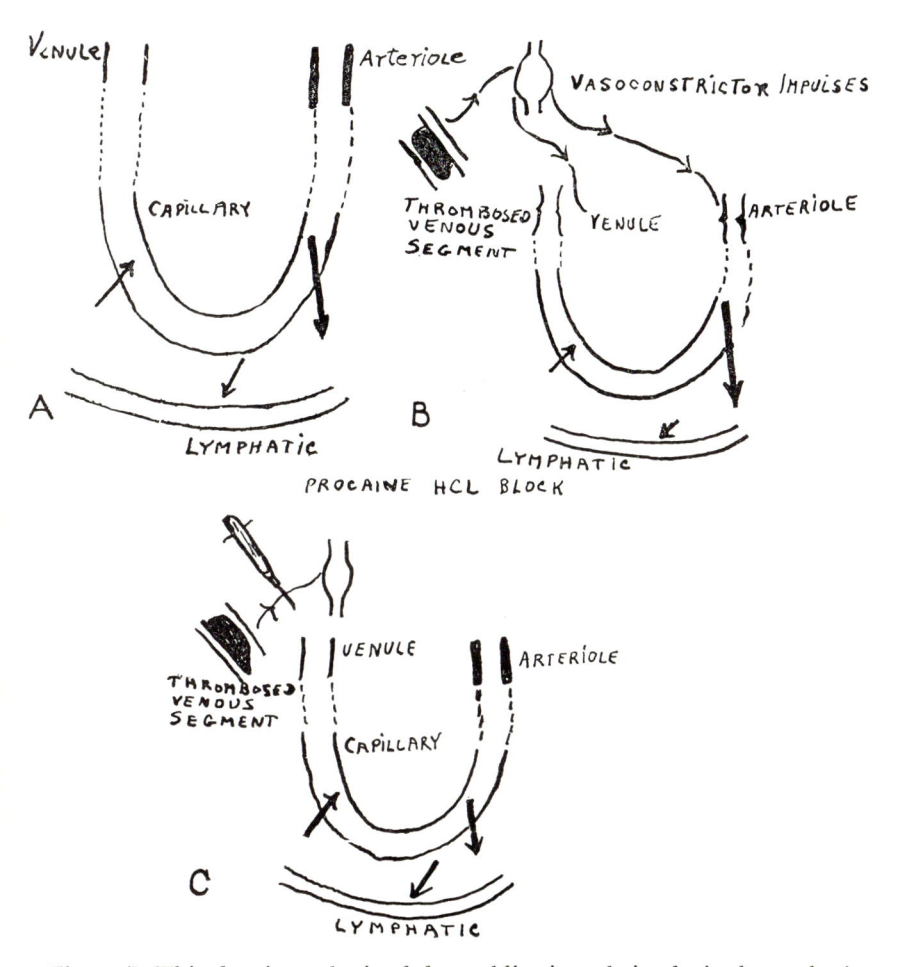

Figure 7. This drawing submitted for publication obviously is the author's attempt at illustration. Functionally, it is almost adequate but lacks clarity of expression. In another sense it is a communication of an idea, sound enough in itself, but needing revision of its "grammar" to convey its meaning.

Halftone Illustrations

The halftone process is used for the reproduction of charts and drawings with gray shading and of photographs—patients, tissues and appearances under the roentgen rays.

The ideal photograph is a perfect print on paper with a glossy

158   *Medical Writing*

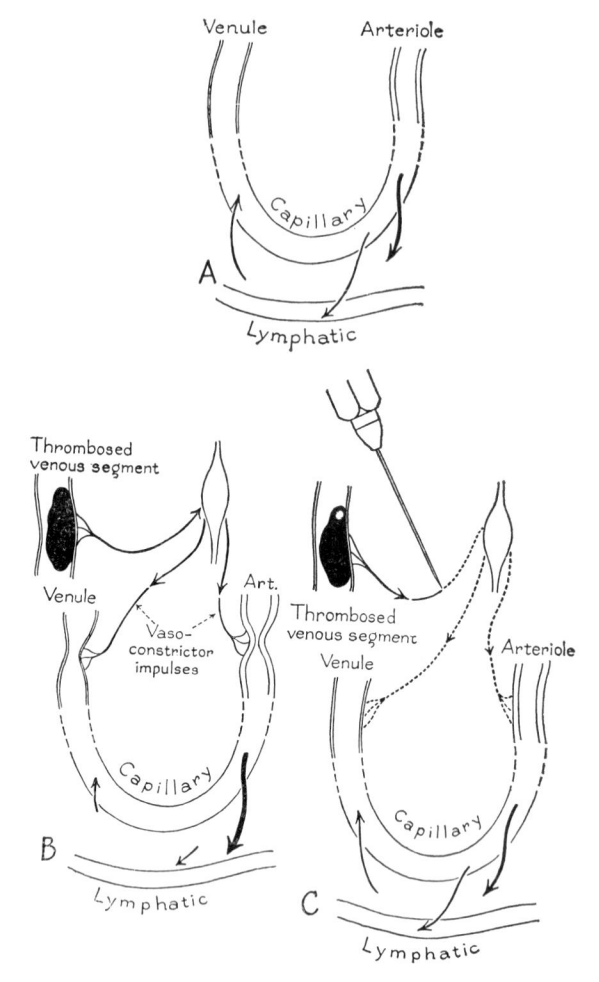

Figure 8. This is the same idea as that in Figure 7, expressed by an experienced artist to whom the original sketch was sent for revision. Crisp, clean lines and legible lettering convey the meaning of the author with the added advantage of a well-planned arrangement to fit the type page. The reader will instinctively put his faith in this useful explanatory diagram.

finish. Tone drawings with few or no hard black lines usually result in good illustrations by the halftone process.

Halftone engravings are made in two major styles: *square-finish cuts*, in which the background is left with its light gray tint made up of tiny dots; and *outlined cuts*, in which the engraver cuts this background away. This latter process is much more expensive, since it is hand work, and if the background contains any lettering, the engraver must work around it very carefully. To escape this the engravers resort to *combination plates* which are actually a combination of two films—one of the halftone, outlined, the other a strong contrast film of the lettering, the two being carefully superimposed and the plate etched. This method, while producing attractive plates, has, besides its added expense of hand work, a very definite hazard, for the illustration's outlines, which may have been soft and hazy in the original, now emerge very sharply contrasted to the white paper and sometimes upset the balance of light and shade which the artist worked hard to achieve. Then, too, the engraver, not being familiar with the subject matter, may unwittingly distort the outlines. (See Fig. 19.)

When unusual contrast is deemed desirable by the author, a method of reproduction called *dropped highlights* can be employed. Cuts made by this method, however, cost three times as much as regular halftones, and the author may be asked to bear part of the costs—in other words, all over and above the cost of regular halftones.

When the photograph is being taken, the camera should be focused on the detail to be shown. Keep prominently in mind that in all probability the picture will have to be reduced for publication; hence an unnecessary expanse of general background, the physician or nurse responsible for the patient, apparatus that has no direct bearing on the condition and similar nonessentials should be eliminated, so that the space available will be devoted not to the background or to the wording but to the object to which attention is called. It is possible to have all unnecessary details airbrushed out by the photographer, but retouching of this kind is expensive and may result in the loss of portions of the picture that are essential or in other modifications that are not desirable.

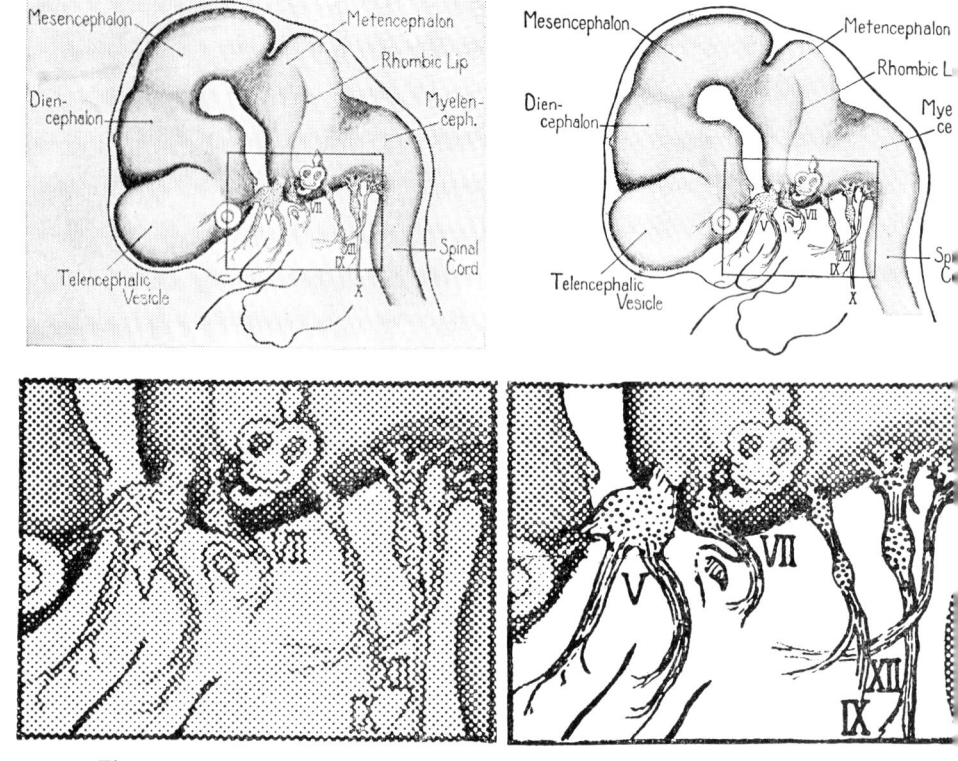

Figure 9. The halftone method of reproduction. (Upper left) Square-finish plate with screen over entire picture, lines and lettering. (Upper right) Combination plate on which the halftone is confined to the picture while the lines and lettering outside are solid black. The engraver has mechanically removed all screen from the background before superimposing the black film over the halftone film prior to etching. (Lower left) An enlargement of the area shown in the rectangle of the square finish plate to show the overall screen. Compare this with the same rectangle enlarged from the combination plate (lower right).

SPECIAL TYPES OF ILLUSTRATIONS

Photomicrographs

If the author has large photomicrographs, before submitting his article for publication he should decide how much they are to be reduced to be accommodated to the page size of the periodical. Some authors prefer to trim their photomicrographs rather than to have the magnification reduced; others desire to show the entire picture and have it brought down to the required size by reduction in the magnification. Consequently, when large photomicrographs are submitted without instructions as to the method by which they are to be reduced to fit the type column, correspondence is entailed and sometimes delay in publication results. The width of the type column of any journal for which an article is intended should be similarly noted. A better appearance will be obtained if illustrations do not exceed that measurement in width or height, although they may be a little larger if this is unavoidable. Notes on magnification should be readjusted after the reproduction size has been decided, but these should never be marked on the photographic print.

Roentgenograms

Roentgenograms should be reproduced as interpreted by the roentgenologist—i.e. with opaque masses white and translucent tissues dark. If a contact print is furnished this order will be reversed, and in addition, important details are lost in the process. Hence a better illustration results if made from the actual film.

In preparing the roentgenogram, the experienced roentgenologist will mark it to identify the essential points. The markings, however, should not be so obtrusive as to mar the effect of the complete reproduction. The points of importance may be suitably identified by the insertion of lines on the roentgen ray film.

To the physician who secures it and to the reader, the roentgen ray photograph is actual evidence of the facts brought out in the case report. If an author is trustworthy and reliable, he need not provide actual evidence for his reader, but he should select his roentgenograms on the basis of new points to be brought out in the specific case. It is unnecessary to include six roentgenograms to illustrate a niche in the stomach as it occurred in six cases unless something distinctly new is to be presented concerning each of these niches. In a paper describing a method of making the ureters, the kidneys or the gallbladder visible by the injection of an opaque substance, it is unnecessary to have more than one or two pictures showing the results of the process. Obviously, the best in the series will be selected. The author may then state in his text that 18 or 20 similar plates were prepared.

SHADING PROCESSES

The Ben Day process—named after the inventor, Benjamin Day—is a process for producing a variety of shaded tints by the use of gelatin films. It is used particularly in connection with zinc line engravings. Unfortunately it must be applied by the photoengraver who must be furnished with complete directions and "guide" sketches. A much simpler method consists of a transparent film on which has been printed a pattern of black dots or lines which is to be attached by rubbing to the area to be shaded and the surplus cut away with a sharp needle. For shading over black areas, white dots or lines are supplied. With this method, shading can be done by any artist directly under the author's supervision.

COLORED ILLUSTRATIONS

The reproduction of illustrations in color is expensive. If possible, some means other than the color process should be devised to depict what it is desired to show. In drawings, for instance, it is possible to use varieties of cross hatching and stippling to differentiate the various portions; the significance of these various forms may be explained in the legend to appear under the illustration.

RETURN OF ILLUSTRATIONS

If the author wishes his illustrations returned, the word "Return," together with his address, should be written on the label on each picture, and in submitting his manuscript the author should specifically request the return of the illustrations after publication. It is necessary that illustrations be held by the publisher until the article is in pages, so that they may be properly identified by the proofreaders.

SUMMARY OF RULES PERTAINING TO ILLUSTRATIONS

1. Illustrations must illustrate.
2. Illustrations should be correctly numbered and identified. On the mounting of each the author should indicate the top

and give his name and the number of the illustration. This is done preferably by means of a paper label pasted on.
3. Illustrations should be sent flat—never rolled or folded.
4. Indication should be made in the margin of the manuscript at the place where the author would like to have each illustration inserted.
5. Expense can be saved by grouping illustrations when this is feasible. Such groups should be published as text figures, not as plates, and the individual sections should be lettered instead of numbered.
6. Lettering on illustrations should appear, preferably, within the borders of the picture.
7. Because the cost of reproducing illustrations is such an important item, authors may be requested to assume part or all of the expense of publishing illustrations in color as well as the cost of reproducing what it considers more than a reasonable number of black and white illustrations. The cost of reproducing illustrations in society transactions must be borne by the author or by the society.

CONCLUSIONS

Suitable illustrations attract the interest of a reader and, if well selected and properly reproduced, are likely to cause more readers to familiarize themselves with the contents of an article than would otherwise notice it. Obviously, the eye is caught by the picture even before the reader's attention is attracted by the title or by the text. Moreover, illustrations can constitute actual scientific evidence. Their preparation should be given meticulous attention. In this connection, the following paragraph from the preface of S. Ramón y Cajal's "Histologie du système nerveux de l'homme et des vertébrés"[1] is interesting:

> Illustrations, some in black and white and others in color, clarify the text of this volume; their number is considerable. There are never enough illustrations, especially in works on anatomy, in which, it might be said, the illustrations are more necessary than the text—on one condition, it is true, that they are, like ours, copied with the most

[1] Ramón y Cajal, S.: Histologie du système nerveux de l'homme et des vertébrés. Paris, A. Maloine, 1909.

scrupulous attention to detail from irreproachable preparations. Such illustrations are nature itself, the facts themselves, to be submitted to examination and free interpretation by a host of observers. They are likewise documents of infinite value to which future generations can have recourse in the continuous struggle of opinions and theories. The text itself represents the author—that is, one of many ways of looking at nature and facts—with his unavoidable tendency to twist and simplify according to the ineradicable conditions of his mental processes.

14
TABLES AND CHARTS

G RAPHIC METHODS of presentation add greatly to the interest of scientific papers. Through tables and charts, almost at first glance the reader may obtain an understanding of the salient features that he might secure only with difficulty from the complete text.

TABLES

Data should be tabulated only when it is possible to present them more vividly in that form than in the text. An unwieldy table is likely to be studied by few readers. As tabular matter usually is handled on a separate typesetting machine, each table should be typewritten on a separate sheet of paper, with the author's name on either the front or the back. The tables may then be given to the compositor without delaying the prepartion of the other material. For the sake of appearance, it is desirable that a uniform style be followed in tables. If there is more than one table, they should be numbered consecutively, and each should have a descriptive heading. A typical heading is as follows:

TABLE 3
DISTRIBUTION OF PATIENTS ACCORDING TO AGE

The headings of the vertical columns should indicate the subjects chiefly concerned. The variations should be indicated in the left-hand column, in which can be given the period of the various observations or the record number of the animals, cases or other objects to be contrasted. In other words, the vertical columns contain the like data.

Table can almost always be condensed. Often a factor that is common to all entries in a column can be incorporated in the heading of the column, thus saving space. A column that contains no variable factors may be eliminated and the important point covered by a footnote to the table. When there are only one or two variations in 25 or 30 items, frequently it is possible to use a footnote for each of the cases that vary.

Footnotes to tables usually are indicated by asterisks, daggers and similar reference marks, rather than by numbers. The usual sequence of the symbols is *, †, ‡, §, ||, ¶ and #. If additional symbols are needed, those just listed may be doubled. In inserting footnotes one should take those needed in the heading of the columns first and then those in the body of the table, working from left to right and downward. The accompanying table illustrates the use of headings and footnotes.

TABLE 6
CAUSES OF DEATH IN CASES OF DIABETIC COMA

	Fatalities in Hospitals in Rochester	Fatalities Elsewhere*	Total
Uncomplicated diabetic coma	3	8	11
Cardiovascular disease	4	1	5
Pneumonia and its complications	2	2	4
Bilateral pyelonephritis with metastatic abscesses	1	..	1
Septicemia	1	..	1
Erysipelas	1	..	1
Acute yellow atrophy and toxic nephrosis (arsenical?)	1	..	1
Hodgkin's disease	1	..	1
Hemochromatosis	1	..	1
Diabetic gangrene	1	..	1
Advanced pernicious anemia and coma	1	..	1
Carcinoma (sigmoid flexure)	..	1	1
Meningitis, tuberculous (?)	..	1	1
Acute pancreatitis†	..	1	1
Addison's disease†	..	1	1
Intestinal hemorrhage from unknown cause	..	1	1
Heat prostration	..	1	1
Cause unknown	..	5	5
Totals	17‡	22§	39

*Cities listed in the text.
†Diagnosis verified by necropsy elsewhere.
‡Diagnosis verified by necropsy in 14 cases.
§Accurate records of confirmation of diagnosis at autopsy not available.

For purposes of condensation it sometimes is desirable to use abbreviations which it would be undesirable to employ in the text. Standard abbreviations should be employed when they exist. If unusual abbreviations are used, they should be explained in a footnote to the table. (A list of standard abbreviations used in medical and scientific literature appears in Chapter 8.)

In preparing a table the author should bear in mind the size of the page of the periodical in which it is to appear. It is to the advantage of both the author and the reader to have the table prepared so that it may stand upright; rarely does an editor arrange for the insertion of a broadside table—one on its side. When statistical data cannot be presented in any other manner, it is possible to make exceedingly large tables, which are folded and inserted in the periodical after the forms are assembled. This, however, is a costly hand process, and it is customary for periodicals to ask authors to bear the extra expense entailed. In special instances arrangements are made to spread a table across two facing pages, thus avoiding duplication of material. This likewise is not generally desirable, as it involves difficulty in arranging the article in consecutive order in the pages.

As in the case of illustrations or, in fact, of any material that has previously been published, written permission must be secured from the copyright holder if a table is reproduced from some other periodical. The table should be reproduced as nearly in the form of the original as typographic facilities permit, and the fact that it is taken from another source may be indicated in a footnote.

CHARTS

Lines in charts should be differentiated by their composition rather than by the use of different colors. They may be heavy or light, continuous or broken (composed of long or short dashes; of dots; of dots and dashes; or of dots, circles and dashes). (See Fig. 10). A scatter graph may also be used.

Much of the paper sold for charting purposes has blue, green, brown or light red cross rulings, which ordinarily are not of the same intensity and which in reproduction give a spotted and broken appearance. Usually only every fifth or tenth line is required as a coordinate in locating the points that determine the path of the curve; hence chart paper without the intermediate lines—that is, with large squares—or chart paper in which the in-

168   *Medical Writing*

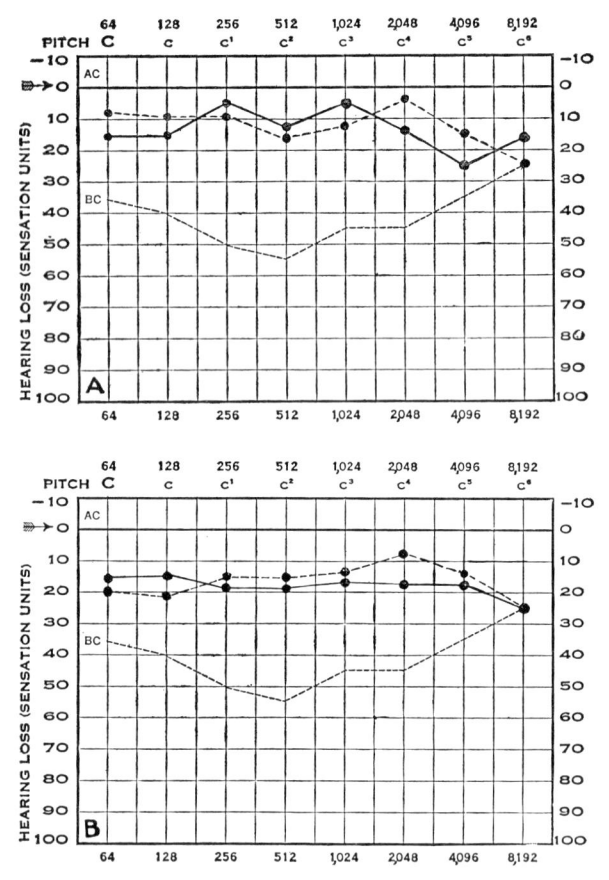

Figure 10. These audiograms (A taken before and B taken after the administration of procaine hydrochloride) illustrate the use of different kinds of lines. The two lines emphasized with dots show the record for the patient; the solid line shows that for the right ear and the broken line shows that for the left. The broken line below shows the audiometer readings for a person with normal hearing.

termediate lines are light blue and can be dropped in reproduction is preferable.

Charts should be condensed as much as possible to permit reproduction with the least possible reduction. Waste space is avoided by bringing the borders down or up close to the curves at all points and by eliminating from the surface of the chart unimportant or irrelevant data. If a temperature curve ranges from 97 to 104° F, it is unnecessary to reproduce the whole of a temperature chart made to show variations from 95 to 107° F. The temperature chart ordinarily used for the hospital record does not reproduce as satisfactorily as the chart prepared particularly to show the temperature, with the varying degrees indicated by printed letters on the left-hand margin. Unless neatly printed, words and sentences placed on the face of the chart spoil its appearance; therefore, it usually is better to place letters, numerals, asterisks or other indicating devices on the face of the chart and to explain them in the legend. All letters, numbers and symbols on charts should be sufficiently large to permit reduction necessary to accommodate the chart to the type column. Frequently papers are accompanied by charts so large that they require well over 50 per cent reduction, but the numbers and letters thereon will not permit more than 5 per cent reduction. Such charts must be returned to the author to be redrawn, which may occasion delay in publication.

Figures 11 and 13 show amateurish charts received for publication and figures 12 and 14 show the same charts after the editor had them redrawn for the author.

The same rules apply in the presentation of statistical data by the use of various shadings. Shading should be done in black and white rather than in colors. For the purpose of contrast, solid black squares may be placed next to white squares or next to squares filled with dots, with oblique lines or with circles. It is the rule of practically all periodicals that the author shall be asked to bear the extra expense of reproducing in color charts in which the data could be presented as well in black and white.

170　　　　　　　　　　*Medical Writing*

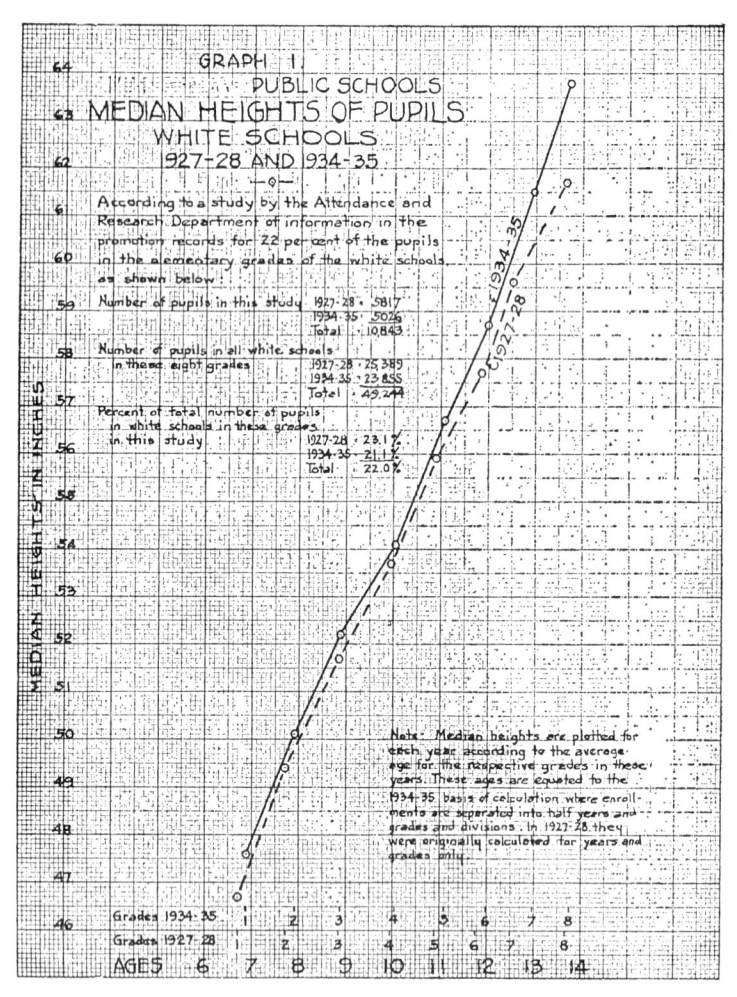

Figure 11. A reproduction of a chart as submitted by the author. The blurred background makes it difficult to read the letters and figures and to follow the curves and gives the chart an unpleasant appearance.

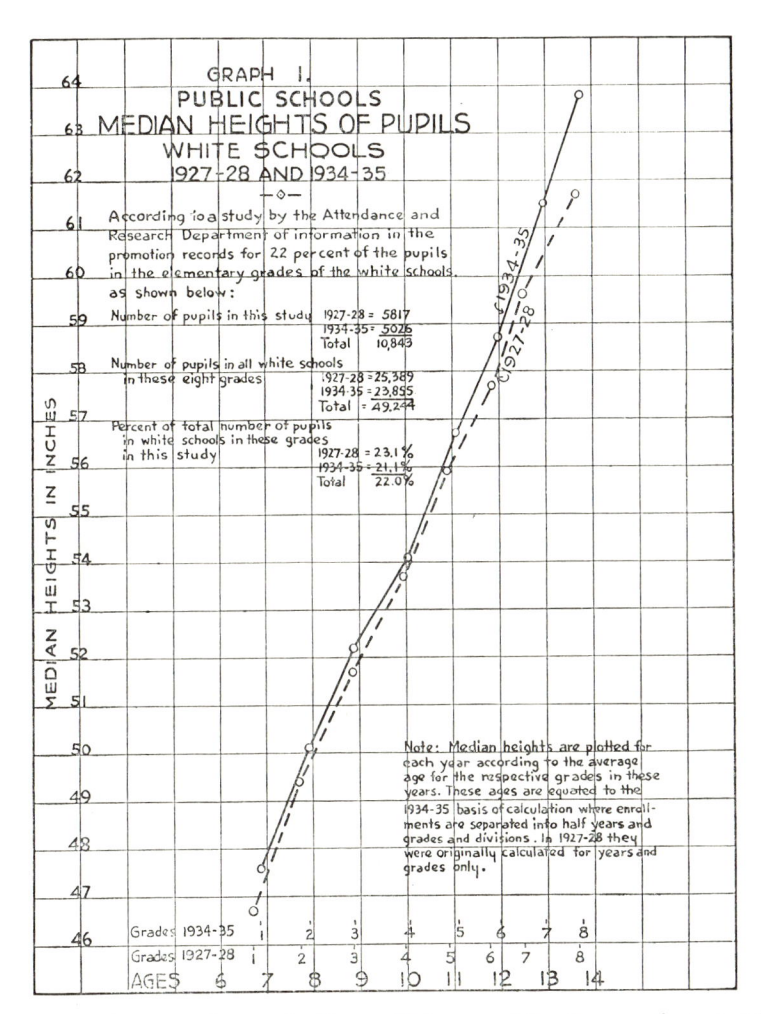

Figure 12. The same chart as in Figure 11 improved by the use of paper with simple, large squares. It might be improved further by elimination of some of the statistical data, which could be included in the legend, in the text or in a table.

172   *Medical Writing*

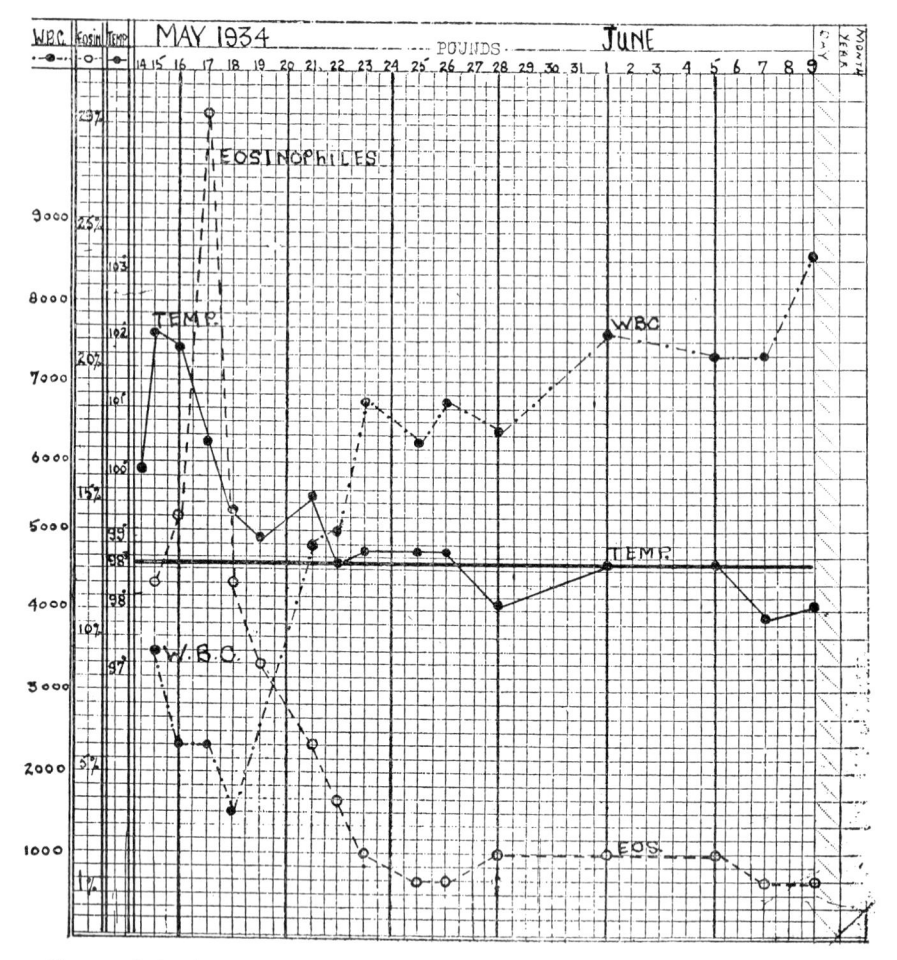

Figure 13. Broken lines in the background give this chart a spotted and unattractive appearance; crooked and illegible letters and crowded and indistinct figures prevent it from conveying the author's information to the reader.

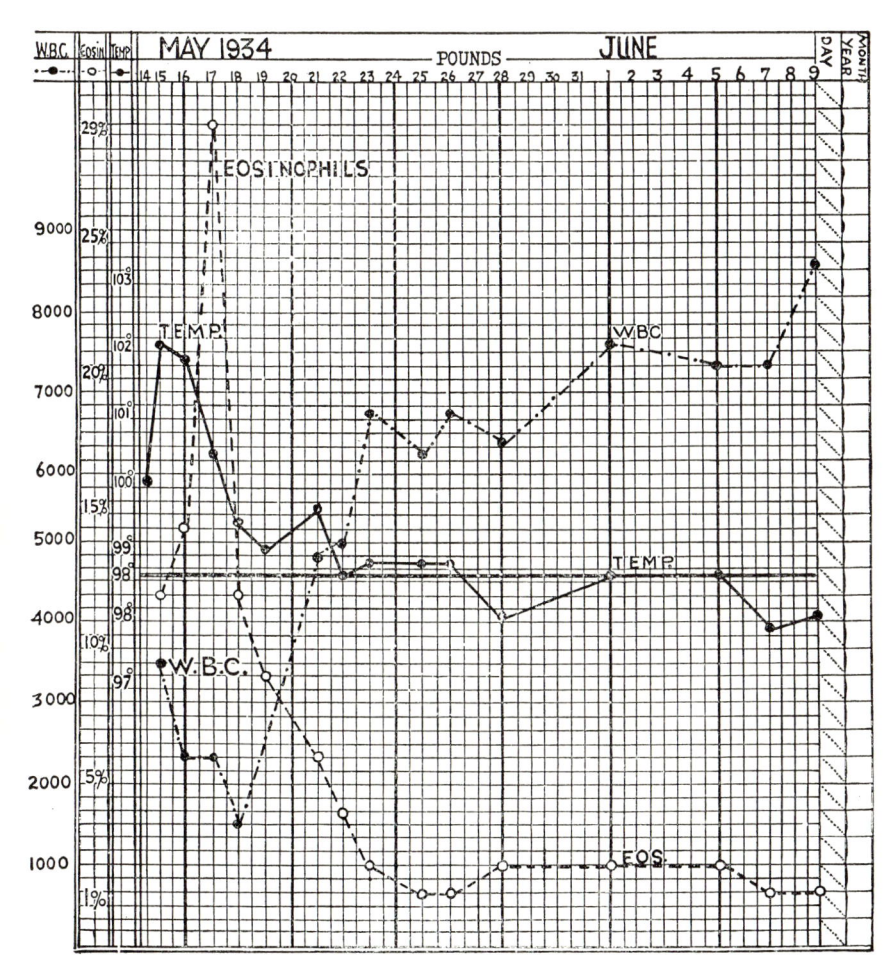

Figure 14. Clean, well-printed chart paper, careful lettering and enlarged figures have improved the chart shown in Figure 13.

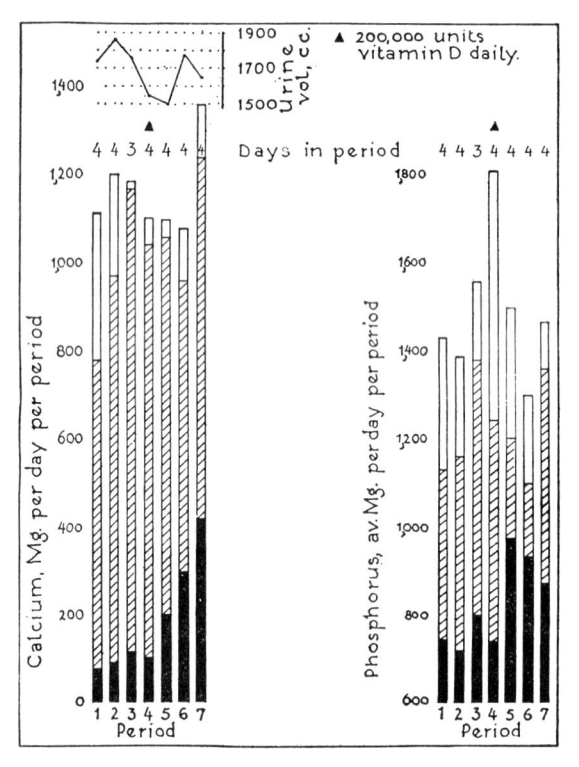

Figure 15. This chart illustrates the use of different kinds of shading.

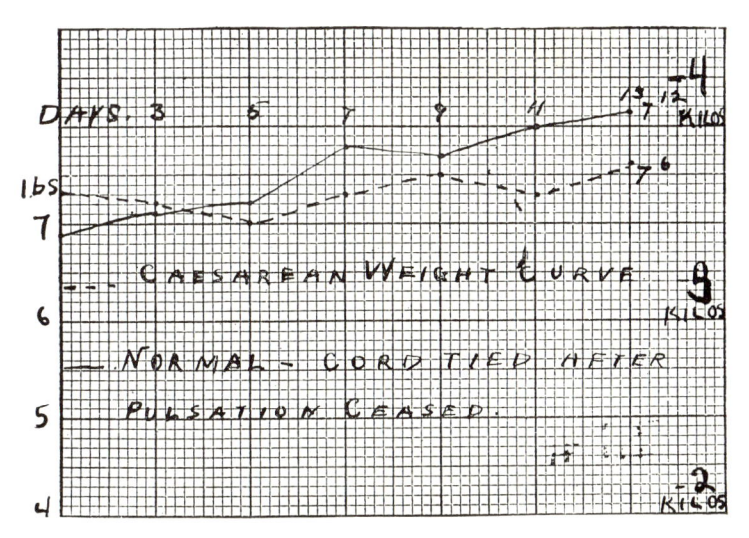

Figure 16. The chart paper on which this chart was made was ruled in green. Such paper is pleasing to the eye in the original but gives an uneven and smudgy effect in the black-and-white reproduction. The excessive amounts of background and of wording, moreover, distract attention from the curves themselves.

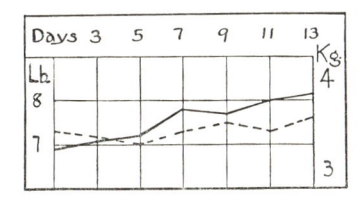

Figure 17. The chart shown in Figure 16 redrawn on chart paper ruled in black, with larger squares. It occupies less space than the original, is more pleasing to the eye and is easier to read. The explanation of the lines would appear in the legend.

15
REVISION OF THE MANUSCRIPT

IN HIS WELL-WRITTEN, interesting and practical book entitled *Notes on the Composition of Scientific Papers,* Sir. T. Clifford Allbutt[1] said that it was his custom to make at least four drafts of a manuscript before it could be considered ready for the printer. The first draft was compiled from notes that had been carefully collected on slips and arranged in logical order. Redundant words, phrases, sentences and paragraphs were then deleted, resulting in the shortening of the manuscript from 20 to 25 per cent, and sentences out of position or coherence or logical development of thought were moved to better positions. Naturally, also, second thoughts (in many instances better than first thoughts) were inserted as they occurred.

In the next revision, sentences and paragraphs were recast so as to carry but one meaning; ornamental and figurative passages were modified or removed, and particular attention was given to the choice of exact words for the meanings to be conveyed. After a few weeks had elapsed, Sir Clifford again read the entire manuscript with refreshed attention, making final additions and revisions.

Consider now how the average manuscript is written. The physician surrounds himself with textbooks, reprints, periodicals and penciled notes and starts to write his paper—probably in longhand. After more or less worry and possibly some sleepless nights, he breathes a sign of relief, thanks heaven that it is finished and

---

[1]Albutt, T. Clifford: *Notes on the Composition of Scientific Papers,* 3rd ed. London, Macmillan, 1923.

has it typewritten. He may read the typewritten copy and make one or two corrections before sending it to a medical journal; more likely, he reads the paper before a society and then, without any revision worthy of the name, sends it for publication. Not a few manuscripts offered for publication bear evidence that the only reading given them was that of the typist and that she did not correct her own misspelling. "To have a manuscript typewritten," said an editorial writer in the *British Medical Journal,* "and then to send it for publication without revision is a crime comparable to operating with unwashed hands."

Many physicians have envied Sir William Osler his easy command of English in his writing. In his library is a collection of some of his manuscripts, showing the various stages in their preparation. First are notes on paper of various kinds, evidently written on trains and at opportune moments; then a rough outline in longhand; next the first typewritten copy, with interlineations, transpositions and deletions; then the second typewritten copy, which also bears evidence of much modification, and, finally, a third typewriten copy, which evidently was used by the printer. Even this last copy has a few minor corrections.

Anatole France, Nobel prize winner in literature, said that seven revisions are necessary, and that an eighth is desirable in order to make sure that the corrections on the seventh have been understood. "In the first," it has been said, "he enlivened what had been platitudinous. The second was for 'weeding out the dandelions,' whos, whiches and whoms. In the third, he eliminated the semicolons, shortened his sentences and struck out phrases which merely linked one sentence with another or marked a transition from one thought to another, a task that should not be left to the reader. In the fourth draft he gave special attention to the order of sentences and to the repetition of the same word; he looked on the recurrence as a warning to rewrite the sentence, not to search for a synonym. The fifth draft saw the disappearance of adjectives, for he was of the opinion of Voltaire that, though the adjective might agree with the substantive in gender, number and case, often it did not suit it. From the sixth draft he chipped away what he called the pastry, all that was adventitious and redundant, and over the seventh draft he passed the plane, for, he said, 'a good writer is like a good cabinet maker—he planes his phrases smooth.' "

Trelease and Yule,[2] in their practical book entitled *Preparation of Scientific and Technical Papers*," suggest 10 revising processes, pointing out, however, that it is neecssary to recopy the pages only after they have become crowded with corrections. Their first revision is for consistency, involving the removal of irrelevant material and the avoidance of contradictions. Next, the structure of individual sentences is improved, and it is emphasized that few sentences should have more than 30 words. The punctuation should be simple. Revisions are then made for clearness of sentences and paragraphs; to avoid repetition; to justify the use of conjunctions, interjections and relative pronouns; to make certain that the article reads smoothly; to correct punctuation; to make the use of capitals and italics and the subheadings consistent and last, to make certain that statements are accurate.

An article appearing in a state medical journal apparently was published without revision; it presented most of the faults mentioned in this book, as well as many of those referred to in elementary books on grammar and rhetoric. The entire essay comprised 2,800 words. It was divided into 12 paragraphs, and contained only 33 sentences—an average of 84 words to a sentence. One paragraph, consisting of a single sentence of 208 words, read:

> We know, of course, that a few of the state societies have recently taken it upon themselves to initiate a campaign intended to counteract in some measure the ravages of quackery and such an effort is a very praiseworthy one and we bespeak for it a considerable degree of success, and it behooves us as members of the societies to assist in every possible manner the furtherance of this effort, and also seek to enlist the aid of those of the profession who are not yet members of our societies, that a united front may be presented in the fight as this is essential to the success of the campaign and we must realize further, that such a united effort does not at all excuse an individual effort but rather makes this more obligatory and should remember also, that in this as in all other campaigns of any character, that we will get only as much out of it as we put into it, so there must be no shirking of our obvious duty in this regard.

---

[2]Trelease, S. F. and Yule, E. S.: *Preparation of Scientific and Technical Papers*, 3rd ed. Baltimore, Williams & Wilkins, 1937.

Revision of Manuscript

The first step in revision included the bracketing of unnecessary words and the breaking up of the long sentences into several short ones. The revised paragraph is shown in Figure 18.

> [We know, of course, that] a few of the state societies have recently [taken it upon themselves to] initiated a campaigns [intended] to counteract [in some measure] the ravages of quackery. [and] such an effort is [a very] praiseworthy, [one and we bespeak for it a considerable degree of success,] and it behooves [us as] members of the societies to assist in every possible manner. [the furtherance of this effort, and] *They should* [also seek to enlist the aid of] ~~those~~ *physicians* [of the profession] who are not yet members of ~~our~~ *the* societies, that a united front may be presented. [in the fight as] this is essential to the success of the campaign. [and we must realize further, that] such a united effort does not [at all] excuse [an] individual effort but [rather] makes this [more] obligatory. [and should remember also, that] in this as in all [other] campaigns [of any character, that] we will get only as much (out) [of it] as we put into it, so. there must be no shirking of [our] obvious duty. [in this regard.]

Figure 18. The first step in revision.

When the paragraph was copied after revision, it appeared as follows:

> A few of the state societies have recently initiated campaigns to counteract the ravages of quackery. Such an effort is praiseworthy, and it behooves members of the societies to assist in every possible manner. They should also seek to enlist the aid of physicians who are not yet members of the societies, that a united front may be presented. This is essential to the success of the campaign. Such a united effort does not excuse individual effort but makes this obligatory. In this as in all campaigns we will get out only as much as we put in. There must be no shirking of obvious duty.

With further revisions for punctuation, diction and emphatic style, the paragraph appeared as in Figure 19.

> A few ~~of the~~ state societies have recently initiated ^praiseworthy campaigns to counteract the ravages of quackery. ~~Such an effort is praiseworthy, and~~ it behooves *the* members ~~of the societies~~ to assist in every possible manner. They should ~~also~~ seek to enlist the aid of physicians who are not yet members, ~~of the societies,~~ that a united front may be presented. This is essential to the success of the campaign. ^however, ~~Such a~~ united effort, (does not excuse *one from* individual effort but makes ~~this~~ *it* (obligatory. In this, as in all campaigns, *one* ~~we~~ will get out only as much as (*one puts*) ~~we put~~ in. There must be no shirking of obvious duty.

Figure 19. The appearance of the material in Figure 18 after further revision.

Here, then, is the paragraph as finally revised, probably still susceptible of improvement in diction:

> A few state societies have recently initiated praiseworthy campaigns to counteract the ravages of quackery. It behooves the members to assist in every possible manner. They should seek to enlist the aid of physicians who are not yet members, that a united front may be presented. This is essential to the success of the campaign. United effort, however, does not excuse one from individual effort but makes it obligatory. In this, as in all campaigns, one will get out only as much as one puts in. There must be no shirking of obvious duty.

16
PROOFREADING

Nearly all periodicals submit proof to the author prior to publication. It is then his privilege and duty to scrutinize the proof—whether in galley or page form—to make certain that the printed article which will appear under his name is entirely to his satisfaction. When an article has been prepared by more than one author, proof will be sent to the one whose name appears first, in the absence of written directions to the contrary. On special request, proof may be sent to each of the several authors.

CORRECTIONS

Reading proof will be facilitated if the following rules are observed:

1. Read the proof against the manuscript, checking carefully for omissions, errors in spelling and fact and other deviations from copy.
2. Never erase or alter any proofreader's marks made on proof.
3. Answer all queries written on proof. Queries are made in the interest of accuracy and not in a spirit of criticism. (Sometimes they are set in large type, called "catchlines," intended to catch the author's attention.) Cross out the question mark or draw a line through the catchline and correct the questioned portion if it is wrong. It is unsatisfactory merely to write "O.K." in the margin, for this may not answer the question, leaving the proofreader in doubt as to whether the original text or the suggested change is O.K.

4. Make all corrections legibly in the margin of the proof—never inside the type page or on the manuscript. Do not draw lines from the point at which corrections are to be made into the margin of the proof, for they create confusion; instead, mark your corrections in the margin parallel to the line of type in which the correction is to appear.
5. Put a caret inside the type page at the point where an insertion is to go, but do not put a caret in the margin under the material to be inserted.
6. Use ink of a color different from that already used on the proof. This is to differentiate between your changes and those made by the printer.
7. Use the universally accepted proofreader's signs and symbols as illustrated on pages 184 and 186.
8. When making changes in proof, whenever possible provide space for new words by omitting the same number of letters in closely adjacent material. This will result in a considerable saving in the cost of resetting type.
9. Retype extensive changes on a full-sized sheet of paper, identify the sheet with the galley or page number and paste it firmly to the margin of the proof. Do not use clips or pins.
10. When inserting new material on proof, be sure that the new matter conforms to the style of spelling, punctuation, etc., used in the material already set.
11. Cross out all material to be eliminated.
12. Indicate in the margin where illustrations are to be inserted in the proof. (The publisher, however, reserves the right to digress from your choice if it is unsuitable because of mechanical or economic considerations.)
13. Should you be asked (1) to supply material to add a line or (2) to delete material to eliminate a line, do so carefully in order that the pages may be of the proper depth.
14. Remember that if the type has been set on the linotype machine, a change of as little as one letter or mark of punctuation in a line will necessitate the resetting of the entire line.

Signs Used in Correcting Proof

PARAGRAPHING

¶   Make a new paragraph.
no ¶, or   No paragraph.
run in

INSERTION AND DELETION

the   Insert word, letter or punctuation written in the margin.
Out, see copy   Insert matter omitted.
∧   indicates where insertion is to be made.
𝒅   Delete, or take out, a line or word.

SPACING

\#   Insert space between words, letters or lines.
⌒   Close up, or take out space.
⌒𝒆   Take out let/ter and close up.
⌒\#   Close up, but leave some space.
Center   Put in middle of page or line.

POSITION

↻   Turn to proper position.
⊏   Move to left.
⊐   Move to right.
⊔   Move down a letter, character or word.
⊓   Move up a letter, character or word.
☐   Indent one em.
≡   Straighten a crooked line.
‖   Straighten lateral margin of printing.
tr   Transpose of order words or letters.
tr \#   Transpose space.
✓✓   Correct uneven spacing.
space out   Spread words farther apart.
run over   Run over to next line. (A two letter division is not allowed.)
run back   Run back to preceding line. (Such a division is not allowed.)

Signs Used in Correcting Proof
PUNCTUATION

⊙	Period.
⁐	Comma.
⌄	Apostrophe.
:	Colon.
;	Semicolon.
⌄⌄	Quotation marks.
=	Hyphen (-).
$\frac{1}{en}$	En dash (–).
$\frac{1}{em}$, or ⊢⊣	Em dash (—).
$\frac{2}{em}$	Two em dash (——).
=	Sign of equality (=).
(/)	Parentheses.
[/]	Brackets.

MISCELLANEOUS

⌣	Push down a space that prints.
?	Question to author: Is this right?
stet	Allow to ~~stand~~ as it is.
lc	RESET in lower case.
caps	Reset in capitals.
u	use a capital.
small caps	Reset in small capitals.
rom	Reset in roman.
ital	Reset in italic.
bf	Reset in bold face.
wf	Wrong font (wrong size or style).
∨	Superior figure.
∧	Inferior figure.
×	Type is broken or imperfect.
≡	under a letter or a word indicates capitals.
=	SMALL CAPITALS.
—	*Italics.*
⌇	**Bold face.**
≋	**BOLD FACE CAPITALS.**
≋	**BOLD FACE SMALL CAPITALS.**
⌇	***Bold face italics.***

It was of more than incidental interest to know that the galveston epidmic of last year was accompanied with a scourge of Mosquitoes of/x// or the species (Stegomyia fasciata, or Aedes aegypti) responsible for the the transmission of yellow fever.

It was of more than incidental interest to know that the Galveston epidemic of last year was accompanied by a scourge of mosquitoes of the species (*Stegomyia fasciata*, or *Aedes aegypti*) responsible for the transmission of yellow fever.

Figure 20. Above is a paragraph as corrected by the proofreader; below it is the same paragraph after the corrections have been made.

15. Indicate on galley proof what the running head should be if the title of the article is too long to be accommodated.
16. Never cut master proof apart. If dummying is requested, an extra set will be supplied with instructions.
17. Mark your file set of proof exactly like the master set.
18. Return the printer's master set promptly, together with the manuscript. Meeting scheduled publication dates depends partially on your cooperation in this respect.
19. Use your duplicate set of page proofs to make the index for a book.

The author should remember that the proof has been sent to him for *reading*, not rewriting. Consciousness of this fact will save considerable expense which is often wholly or partially chargeable to the author.

17
INDEXING

In compiling an index, the author should remember that he is constructing a tool intended for one purpose only: to enable the reader *quickly and easily* to find the subject he is interested in. The author already knows the subject matter of his book, but too often he forgets that the reader must depend on a more or less imperfect knowledge of what to seek; therefore index entries should be couched in language understandable to the reader. For example, should the author index all entries pertaining to that subject under the words "Hansen's disease," forgetting the commonly used "leprosy," a reader who may be unfamiliar with the former term may think the subject of leprosy is not discussed.

ORGANIZING THE MATERIAL

Usually the author will receive a duplicate set of page proofs simultaneously with the printer's master set. Before returning the printer's set, he should incorporate every mark thereon into his own set of pages, so that he can retain an exact copy of the proof as released to the printer. He should pay particular attention to any marks indicating transposition of material from one page to another, for this will affect the subsequent pagination and, in turn, the index.

The first step in compiling an index is to check all the pages for proper numerical sequence. Then, using a colored crayon pencil (preferably red), the author should underscore those words, phrases and subjects he wishes to have appear in the index. This procedure should be followed throughout the entire page proof. He need not restrict himself to underlining items in the text only, but may—and should—include center heads and side heads as well as chapter titles. Simultaneously, as he progresses through the page proof, he should note in the margin of the page any cross references that should be accommodated in the writing of the index entries. For example, if "pregnancy" is under discussion, he should write down the synonyms "gestation" and "gravidity." (Later he will choose one of these words under which to group the page references, treating the other words as cross references. See pages 189 and 190.

As a general rule, to be proportionate in length, an index should contain about three times as many entries as there are pages of text indexed—in other words, each page of text will contribute about three entries to the index. By no means is this rule of thumb to be construed as obligatory; it is offered merely as a guide to the author who is endeavoring to build a functional index which tells the story but is free of "padding."

After laying this groundwork, the author is ready for the actual writing of the items which will comprise the index.

WRITING THE ENTRIES

The author may write the entries in longhand, or he may type them (see page 194). In either case, work will be facilitated by using a continuous roll of paper tape such as is used in cash registers. It is of a weight conducive to easy handling and later can be cut apart into separate entries for rearrangement into alphabetical order.

Another useful device is regulation size $8\frac{1}{2}$ by 11 inch paper perforated into 10 parts. Each entry may be written or typed on one of the sections and later the whole can easily be separated into its parts.

Cards measuring 3 by 5 inches are used frequently. These are also available now in rolls, the use of which does away with the inconvenience of inserting each card into the typewriter individually.

The author should decide what is the key word in the phrase previously underscored in red—the word most likely to be sought by the reader. Usually the key word will be a noun. Generally speaking, an index should be composed of noun entries—both main entries and subentries—and not of adjective entries unless (a) such adjectives possess a particular significance (as "catalytic reagents") or (b) the noun is vague (as "hereditary conditions"). For example, suppose on page 80 the phrase "external carotid artery" has been underlined. Since the key word is "artery," the entry should be written "artery, carotid, external, 80." (The inversion of the words "external carotid" permits the later insertion of other subentries under the noun "artery" such as "internal carotid," "anterior cerebral," etc.)

If a subject can be discussed under several key words, the author should enter it under all such words, either with the page reference or with a cross reference to the item he considers most important. Examples follow.

    Bronchopneumonia, 87   Gestation (*see* Pregnancy)
        penicillin in, 88   Gravidity (*see* Pregnancy)
                                       Pregnancy, 206–243

Also:
    Penicillin, 102
        in bronchopneumonia, 88

Since each entry and subentry is written on a separate card or slip, it follows that full information must be given for each one, as they are not in any order when being written. For example, since the entry "muscles" may prove to have more than one subentry, the identifying word "muscles" must appear on every subentry even though it will be eliminated in the final editing (see pages 192 and 193).

Likewise in indexing, the use of verbs and phrases should be avoided in favor of nouns. Examples follow.

Avoid: Streptomycin, administering, 102
Avoid: Streptomycin, how to administer, 102
Use: Streptomycin, administration of, 102

Avoid: Antibiotics, and their use in combating infection, 76-110
Use: Antibiotics, use of, to combat infection, 76–110

When writing the entries, the indexer should try to maintain a uniform style throughout, for an ounce of care in this respect will save a pound of work in the final overall editing of the completed index manuscript. He should write inclusive page folios or numbers in full; e.g., 358–362 (not 358–62), 26–28 (not 26–8). He should also write all entries exactly as they appear in the pages of text, paying particular attention to hyphenation and the spelling of proper names and foreign words.

SPECIAL REFERENCES
References to Illustrations

Index references to illustrations may be differentiated from those pertaining to the text proper by underscoring the page number or folio. (These underscored folios then may be set in either italics or boldface, according to the preference of the publisher.) If this plan is adopted, a line should appear on page 1 of the index to the effect that "Page numbers set in *italics* [or **boldface**] refer to illustrations thereon." Examples follow:

    Morbidity, *78*, 103
    Morbidity, **78**, 103

References to Footnotes and Tables

Index references to footnotes or tables may be expressed by using a lower case "n" (for footnote) or "t" (for table) closed up to the page folio. Examples follow:

    Stomatitis, 38n, 42
    Strabismus, 13, 26t

Cross References

For easy readability, the following style is suggested for simple cross references where no folio is linked to the entry:

    Fever, 38
        enteric (*see* Typhoid)
    Oxytocin (*see* Pitocin)

When an entry pertains not only to a page in the book, but also to another entry, the following style is suggested:

    Riboflavin, 262
        (*See also* Vitamin B_2)

ALPHABETIZING THE ENTRIES

The first step in alphabetizing is to arrange the entries into 26 groups—one for each letter of the alphabet. Then, taking the letter A, and later proceeding in like manner with the other letters of the alphabet, the author should arrange the many main entries, subentries and sub-subentries into alphabetical order, for the time being disregarding an apparent repetition of many of the key words. (This situation will be remedied in the final editing.)

Words which are stems in themselves should precede words containing that stem (e.g., "milk" and all its subentries should precede "milk*ing*" even though the subentries of "milk" start with a letter in the alphabet succeeding "i").

Milk sugar, 56
Milking, 58

Single-word entries should precede compound-word entries containing the same word, as follows:

Milk, testing, 56
Milk proteins, 108

Following is an example combining the above illustrations:

Milk, testing, 56
   turbidity, 54
Milk proteins, 108
Milk sugar, 76
Milking, 58
Milky Way, 98

With the exception of combining forms, hyphenated words and proper names should be treated as separate words, as follows:

Brown, Xavier, 22
Brown-Williams, Henry, 84
Browne, F. T., 100

Cardioneurosis, 95
Cardio-omentopexy, 71 } combining forms treated as one word
Cardiopath, defined, 53

Gram-molecule, 89
Grammole, defined, 65

192 *Medical Writing*

A proper name should precede all terms beginning with that name, and the *'s* in the possessive case should be ignored in alphabetizing eponymic entries, as follows:

Dalton, Peter, 23
Dalton's law, 10
Dalton phenomenon, 82

EDITING THE ENTRIES

After arranging the various items in alphabetical order and numbering them in sequence, the author should read the entire index to see that a consistent style of capitalization and punctuation has been used.

At this time, as illustrated below, he should cross out the superfluous information necessarily included when the various entries were being written. Simultaneously with this crossing out of excess material he should also indicate the proper indention of the various subentries and sub-subentries. One way is to use the conventional em marks as follows:

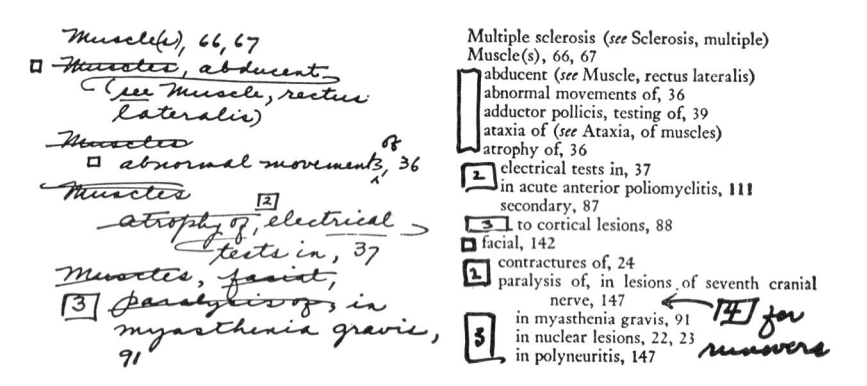

Multiple sclerosis (*see* Sclerosis, multiple)
Muscle(s), 66, 67
  abducent (*see* Muscle, rectus lateralis)
  abnormal movements of, 36
  adductor pollicis, testing of, 39
  ataxia of (*see* Ataxia, of muscles)
  atrophy of, 36
    electrical tests in, 37
    in acute anterior poliomyelitis, 111
    secondary, 87
      to cortical lesions, 88
  facial, 142
    contractures of, 24
    paralysis of, in lesions of seventh cranial nerve, 147
    in myasthenia gravis, 91
    in nuclear lesions, 22, 23
    in polyneuritis, 147

Another way is to employ a series of colored crayon pencil strokes before each entry: one stroke indicating "set flush," two strokes indicating "set one em indent," three strokes indicating "set two ems indent," etc. Lines that run over to a second line (called runovers, overruns or turnovers) should be marked to be indented one em more than the most subordinate entry.

Multiple sclerosis (*see* Sclerosis, multiple)
Muscle(s), 66, 67
abducent (*see* Muscle, rectus lateralis)
abnormal movements of, 36
adductor pollicis, testing of, 39
ataxia of (*see* Ataxia, of muscles)
atrophy of, 36
electrical tests in, 37
in acute anterior poliomyelitis, 111
secondary, 87
to cortical lesions, 88
facial, 142
contractures of, 24
paralysis of, in lesions of seventh cranial
nerve, 147
in myasthenia gravis, 91
in nuclear lesions, 22, 23
in polyneuritis, 147

In both illustrations, representative examples are shown written in longhand, together with their accompanying counterparts as typed. (Obviously these illustrative index samples are the product of the typesetting machine, but the principle remains the same.) Whichever plan is followed, it should be done carefully.

Should there be too few proper names to make a separate "Index of Authors," such names may be incorporated in the "Subject Index" but they may be set in capitals and small capitals to distinguish them from the subject entries. To avoid confusion, all proper names should bear identifying initials or the Christian name if available. For example, "Smith, 452" in an index containing references to other people named Smith would prove of little value to the reader. "Smith, Henry, 452" or "Smith, R. W., 87" is preferable.

In the final editing, the indexer should consolidate on one slip or card, in logical numerical sequence, all entries pertaining to the same key word. For example, if the subject "acromegaly" is discussed in three places in the book (on pages 12, 34 and 56–62, say), in alphabetizing, the indexer will have filed these three separate cards in numerical order. These separate entries should now be converted into one card. The result will read: "Acromegaly, 12, 34, 56–62."

On the other hand, if two or more entries are composed of compound names containing the same preceding modifiers, the compound name should be considered as the main entry and repeated in full. Examples follow:

>Absolute alcohol, 240
>Absolute ether, 309
>Aniline, 34
>>chart of reactions, 36
>>salts of, 38
>
>Aniline black, 40
>Aniline blue, 41

Finally the indexer should check all cross references to eliminate those so-called "dead-end" or "runaround" items that chase the reader fruitlessly from one to another to no purpose. Examples follow:

>Plessimeter (*see* Pleximeter)
>Pleximeter (*see* Plessimeter)

TYPING THE INDEX

After the index has been completely edited, the cards or slips may be submitted for printing or they may be typed in sequence on regular size $8\frac{1}{2}$ by 11 inch paper, thus reducing the overall bulk of the index manuscript. Since errors may creep in during the new typing, the new manuscript must again be read critically, comparing it with the original cards.

The typing should be double spaced, and the indentions of the various subentries should be kept uniform.

INDEX

A

Abbreviations, 108-117
  address, 108-110
    foreign, 109-110
    street, 109
  coined, 31-32
  dates, 111-112
  footnotes, explanations in, 32, 108
  in labels, 153
  miscellaneous, 114-115
  names of persons, 110-111
    titles and degrees, 110-111
  in ophthamology, 113
  organisms, scientific names, 115-116
    bacteria, 115-116
    fungi and parasites, 116
    generic names, other, 116
  prescriptions, 129
    Latin, 129
  rules, miscellaneous, 116-117
  in tables, 32, 166
  weights, measures and time, 112-113
Abstractions in conclusions, 36
Acknowledgment, notes of, 36-37, 59
  contributions
    major, 37, 59
    slight, 37
  footnotes, 37
  support of philanthropies, foundations, and government agencies, 59
  work done in conjunction with others, 60
Adjective
  compound as modifier, 93-97
  endings, variant, 97-99
  modifying word other than one qualified, 55
  as noun, 53-55
Advance, *see* Fee
Agencies, vii

Agent, *see* Editor
Allbutt, Sir T. Clifford, 176
American Chemical Society, 82
  committee of editors of publications, 85
  rules of, 127
American Illustrated Medical Dictionary, 83
American Journal of Psychiatry, 22
American Medical Association
  indexes, 132-133
  publications, vii
  requirements, 19, 57, 62-63, 80, 81, 101, 118
  scientific assembly of, 7
American Medical Directory, 86
American Medical Writers Association, 9
American Roentgenologic Association, 82
American Society of Parasitologists, 82
Anatomic diagnosis in autopsy records, 30
Apothecary measures, *see* Tables and Charts
Army Medical Library, 133-134
Article, *see* Manuscript
Associated Press, 52
Atlantic Monthly, 21-22
Author
  bibliographic references to, 139
  multiple, 59-62
  name, 43-44, 86, 110-111, 144-145
    in indexing, 43-44, 193
    initials, 43
    in foreign publications, 43-44
Autopsy records, 57
  anatomic diagnosis, 30
  negative observations, 30
  research reports, 34

B

BNA, 69, 82
  classical terms, 101
  Latin terms, 82
Bartlett's *Familiar Quotations*, 9
Basle Nomina Anatomica, *see* BNA
Bett, Dr. Walter R., 8
Bibliographic material, 131-142
  citation count, 131-132
  index, 132-133
  references, arrangement and form, 135-138
    bibliographies, 137-138
    footnotes, 135-137
  references, other, vii, 138-142
    form, 140-142
    society proceedings, discussions and legends for illustrations, 138-139
    in tables, 139-140
  securing a bibliography, 132-134
    Current List of Medical Literature, 133-134
    Index-Catalogue of Library of Surgeon General's Office, 134
    Quarterly Cumulative Index Medicus, 133
  securing complete literature, 134-135
  securing medical periodicals, 135
Blakiston's New Gould Medical Dictionary, 83, 86
British Medical Journal, 177
Bureau of Census, 82

C

CIOMS, 68
Capitalization, 106-107
  drugs, trademarked, 127
  lower case, use of, 106-107
  principles, 106
Case report, *see* Subject and Material
Charles, Sir John, 27
Charts, *see* Tables and charts
Citation count, 131-132
Clinical note or suggestion, 33
Conclusions, 34-36
  as fillers, 36
  in framework, 39
Construction of manuscript, 39-45

author's name, 43-44
  faults, 6, 20
  framework, 39
  headings and subheadings, 44-45
  title, 39-43
    ambiguity, 40
    subtitle, 41
  type, 45
    Greek letters and symbols, 45
    italics, 45
Contract, ix
Copyright permission, 37
  from author, 37
  from holder of, 37
  photograph reproduction, 154-155
  release, ix
  written, 37
Corrections
  illustrations, 154
  manuscript preparation, 143-144, 148
  proofreading, 182-186
Cost, 45
  to author, 35, 167, 169
  corrections, 182-186
  illustrations, 149-150, 152, 154, 162
  monograph, 35
  tables, 166
Council for International Organizations of Medical Sciences, *see* CIOMS
Current List of Medical Literature, 133-134

D

Dates, 111-112
  bibliographic references, 111
  descriptions of experiments and cases, 111-112
  numbers, 119
Deadline, ix
Deductions, *see* Conclusions
Diphthongs, 101-102
Directories
  investigators, 86
  physician, 86
Drawings
  diagrammatic line, 33
  halftone, 156-160
  legends, 154

mounting, 151
zinc line, 155-157
see also Illustrations
Dunsany, Lord Edward, 21-22

E

Editing
 principles, 50-51
 professional, 68
 style, 37-38
Editor, 143
 periodical, viii, ix
Enumerations, 125-126
Eponym
 in foreign countries, 70
 hyphenated, 91
 possessive case, 99-101
 table of eponymic diseases, 70-80
 use of, 53, 69-80
Equivalents, *see* Numbers and numbering
Errors, typographic, 37, 144-148
 in quoted material, 37
Essay, 33
Excerpta Medica, 134
Expenses, *see* Cost
Experiments, description of, 34
 dates, 111-112
 numbers, 119

F

Faults, common, 178
 analogous expressions, 52-53
 case report, 30-31
 construction, 6, 20, 39
 duplication
  in monographs, 35
  in research reports, 34
 pharmaceutical nomenclature, 127-128
 tenses, 31
 terminations, 103-105
 terminology, 101
Fee, viii-ix
Fillers, 36
First International Congress on Medical Records, 28
Footnotes
 abbreviations, explanation of, 32, 108
 acknowledgment of contribution, 37
 bibliographic references, 135-137
 dagger or asterisk, use of, 135-136, 166
 index references, 190
 in tables, 166
 typing for publication, 147
Fowler's *Modern English Usage,* 60
Fox, Dr. Howard, 105
France, Anatole, 177
Free-lance writers, viii
Funk and Wagnalls New Standard Dictionary, 83, 87

G

German Anatomical Society, 82
Glossary, 24
Gobbledygook, *see* Terminology
Gould, Dr. George M., 97
Grammar
 correlatives, 17-18
 usage, poor, 14-17
  errors, common, 16-17
   affect and effect, 16
   clauses, restrictive and nonrestrictive, 16-17
Gratitude, expressions of, *see* Acknowledgment, notes of
Greek letters and symbols, *see* Symbols
Gregg, Dr. Allen, 24

H

Halftone illustrations, 156-160
 see also Illustrations
Handbook of Writing, 17
Headings
 center, 44
 index, 187-188
 names in, 116
 side headings, in case reports, 32
 subheadings, 36, 39, 44-45
Hippocratic text, 27
Histologic examination report, *see* Autopsy records
Huneker, James, 8
Hyphen, 88-97
 in compounds, 89-93
 in compound adjective modifiers, 93-97

in names, 43, 91
in symbols, 45

I

Illustrations, 149-164
  colored, 162
  conclusions, 163-164
  index references, 190
  instrument description, accompanying, 32-33
  labeling, 151-154
  legends, 138-139, 147, 154
  permissions, 154-155
  preparation of, 149
    packaging, 151
  reproduction, mediums for, 155-160
    zinc line drawings, 155-157
    halftone, 157-160
  return of, 162
  rules, 162, 163
  shading process, 162
  special types, 160-162
    photomicrographs, 160-161
    roentgenograms, 161-162
Index-Catalogue of the Library of the Surgeon General's Office, 134
Indexes and indexing, 187-194
  alphabetizing entries, 191-192
  author's name, 43-44
  bibliographic references, 131, 134
  citation counts, 131-133
  editing entries, 192-194
  organizing material, 187-188
  periodical, 133-134
  references, special, 190
    cross references, 190
    to footnotes and tables, 190
    to illustrations, 190
  title, 40
  typing index, 194
  writing entries, 188-190
Index Medicus, 133-134
Institute for Scientific Information, 131-132
Instrument, description of, 32-33
International Zoological Congress, 82
Italics, 45

J

Jargon, 47-48
  in foreign countires, 47
  levity, 17-18
Journal of American Medical Association, vii
  index, 132, 134
Journals, *see* Publications

L

Labels
  abbreviations, 153
  cost, 152
  illustration, 150-154
  see also Legends
Lancet (London), 12, 59
Latin prescriptions, 128-130
  abbreviations, 129
Legend, illustration, 138-139, 147, 154
Lettering
  illustration, 151-154, 163
  chart, 169
Letters to the editor, *see* Clinical note or suggestion
Lexicography, 68-69

M

Macdonell, A.G., 12
Manuscript
  bibliographic references to, 131-142
  case report, 27-32
  conclusions, 35-36
  construction, *see* Individual heading
  essay type, 33-34
    addresses, presidential, 33-34
    discussions, 33-34
    forecasts, 33-34
  final copy, 37
  length of, vii, viii, 35
  monograph, 35
  obsolescence, 131
  preparation, *see* individual heading
  proofreading, 182-186
  quoted material, 37-38
  rejection, 3-6
    appearance, as a cause, 143, 150-151
  report of research, 34
    autopsy reports, 34

clinical records, 34
  experiments, 34
  revision, 176-181
  subject and material, 26-38
  summary, 35-36
  types of, 26-27
Material, see Subject and material
Measures
  abbreviations, 112-115
  numbers, 118-119
  values, equivalent, 121-125
    metric, 121-125
    prescriptions, 129
    tables, see Individual heading
  see also Weights, measures and time
Medical, see names of the subjects with which they deal: e.g., Publications, Terminology
Medical Terminology and Lexicography, 68
Medicaments, see Pharmaceutic products and prescriptions
Medlars index, 133-134
Mercier, Charles A., 63
Monograph, 35
  references to, 141
Mycology, 80
  abbreviations, 115-116

N

Names
  abbreviations, 108-117
    cities, 108-109
    organisms, scientific, 115-116
    persons, 110
    states, 108
    streets, 109
  adjective modifier, use as, 100-101
  author's, 43-44, 86, 144-145
  geographic, 87, 108-110
  hyphenated, 91
  in index, 193
  misspelled, frequently, 86
  pharmaceutic products, 127-130
    drugs, trademarked, 127
  possessive case with proper names, 99-101
  spelling, 86

National Association of Science Writers, Inc., viii
National Conference on Nomenclature of Disease, 82
National Medical Library, 133-134
Nomenclature, official codes of, 82
Notes on the Composition of Scientific Papers, 176
Numbers and numbering
  chart, 169
  conclusions, 36
  enumerations, 125-126
  equivalent values, 121-125
    metric, 121-125
  examples, miscellaneous, 120-121
  index, 187
  pagination, 142
  preparation of manuscript, 147-148
  rules, specific, 118-120
    fraction, 118-120
    spell out, 119-120
  in tables, 165
  for typesetter, 45

O

On the Art of Writing, 11-12
Osler, Sir William, 177
Outline, scientific, vii, viii
  in construction, 39
  in monograph, 35

P

Paper, acceptable, 3-7
  rejection, causes for, 3-6
    fancies *vs* facts, 4-5
    material, plethora of one subject, 3-4
    medical society address, 5-6
      deficiencies and success of, 5
    space, lack of, 3
  a standard, 6-7
  types, 26-27
  see also Manuscript
Periodicals, vii, viii
  bibliographic references to, 139-140
  capitalization rules, 106-107
  citation count, 132
  journals, 68

200 *Medical Writing*

library collection, 134
monograph, 35
  publication of, 35
  securing, 135
  style, 83
  see also Publications
Pharmaceutic products and prescriptions, 127-130
  abbreviations, 117
  endocrine and pharmaceutic nomenclature, 127-128
  equivalent values, 122-125
    tables, apothecaries, 122-125
  prescriptions, 128-130
  trademarked drugs, 127
Pharmacopeia of the United States, 127
Photograph
  instrument, 32-33
  legends, 154
  mounting, 151
  reproduction, permission, 154-155
  see also Illustrations
Photomicrographs, 160-161
Phrases, *see* Words and phrases
Plagiarism, 135
Plurals
  English, accepted, 102-103
  foreign, as yet retained, 103
Pocket Oxford Dictionary, 58
Practical paragraph, *see* Clinical note or suggestion
Prefixes, 88
Preparation of manuscript, 50-51, 143-148
  author's name, 144-145
  neatness, 144
  original and carbon copies, 143-144
  paper, 143
  rules, general, 145-148
Preparation of Scientific and Technical Papers, 178
Prescriptions, *see* Pharmaceutic products and prescriptions
Pronouns
  ambiguous, 58-62
  gender, 69
  personal, 60
  plural, 60-61

Proof and proofreading, 182-186
  corrections, 182-186
  signs used in, 184-186
Publication, of manuscript
  articles, 3
  competition, viii
  date of, ix
  description of instrument, 33
  medical society addresses, 5
  preparation of manuscript for, 143-148
Publications
  appearance requirements, 143-148
  bibliographic references, 131
  illustrations, 149
  spelling, reforms, 97
  types of articles, 26
  see also Individual headings, periodicals
Pusey, Dr. William Allen, 63

Q

Quarterly Cumulative Index, 133-134
Quarterly Cumulative Index Medicus, 133-134
Quiller-Couch, Sir Arthur, 8, 11-12
Quoted material, ix, 37-38
  copyrights, 37
  foreign, 69
  trademarked drugs, 127
  typing for publication, 147

R

Reader, 4, 149
References
  bibliographic, *see* Individual heading
  footnote, 135-137
  form, 140-142
  index, 190
  literary, 34
  in society proceedings, discussions and legends for illustrations, 138-139
  source, main, *see* Medlars index
  in tables, 139-140
Register of Articles, *see* Current List of Medical Literature
Rejection of manuscript

Index

causes, 3-6
   appearance, 143
   illustrations, 150-151
Reprints, author's, 37
   see also Copyright
Reproduction, *see* Illustrations
Research report, 34
Review of literature, 33, 60-61, 135
Reviewer, ix
Revision, manuscript, 176-181
   corrections, 143-144, 148, 177-178
   modification, 176
   shortening, 176
Roentgenograms, 161-162

S

Science Citation Index, 131-132
Scientific Assembly of American Medical Association, standards, 7
Shading, illustration
   chart, 169
   processes, 162
Side headings, *see* Headings
Singer, Dr. Charles, 26, 34
Slang, *see* Jargon
Smith's Edwin, Surgical Papyrus, 27
Solecisms, 46-58
   see also Words and phrases
Spelling, 83-105
   classical terminology, 101-105
      diphthongs, 101-102
      plurals, 102-103
      terminations, 103-105
   division of words into syllables, 87-88
   geographic names, 87
   hyphenation, 88-97
      compounds, 89-93
      in compound adjective modifiers, 93-97
   names of persons, 86
      foreign names, 140
   numbers, 118-119
   possessive with proper names, 99-101
      possessive of names ending in sibilant, 101
   simplified, 85-86
   usages, special, 83-85
   variant endings of adjectives, 97-99

Standard Nomenclature of Diseases and Operations, 70, 82
Stenographer's record in autopsy reports, 30
Style, 8-25, 28
   acquiring good style, 24-25
   case report, 28
   correlatives, 17-18
   editing, 37
   fine or fancy writing, 8-11
      hyperbole, 11
      literary allusions, 9
      violations against, 11
   grammar, poor, 14-17
      common errors, 16-17
   gobbledygook, 22-24
   italics, 45
   keeping same point of view, 18-20
      singular and plural forms, 19-20
      tenses, 18-19
   narrative, 28
   nouns used as adjectives, 20-22
   prescriptions, 128
   slang, 17-18
      see also, Jargon
   spelling, 83
   tables, 165
   verbosity, 11-14
      deletions, 11
      space takers or "running start," 12
Subheading, *see* Headings
Subject and material, 26-38
   acknowledgment, notes of, 36-37
   types of articles, 27
      case report, 27-32
      clinical note or suggestion, 33
      complete consideration of a single disease, 34-35
      description of instrument, 32-33
      essay, 33-34
      monograph, 35
      research report, 34
      review of literature, 33
   quoted material, 37-38
      copyrights, 37-38
   summary and conclusions, 35-36
Subtitle, *see* Title
Summary, 34-36, 39

Symbols, 45
  chart, 169
  Greek letters, 45
  mathematical, 45
  minus signs, 45
  in tables, 114, 166
  in footnotes, 166

T

Tables and charts, 165-175
  abbreviations, 114, 115, 166
  charts, 167-175
  headings, 165-166
  numbers, 119
  presentation, 165
  references, 139-140
  research report, 34
  typing for publication, 147
  values, equivalent, 122-125
    area, measures of, 125
    capacity, apothecaries and metric measures of, 124
    capacity, measures of, 125
    length, measures of, 124-125
    weights, apothecaries' and metric, 123-124
    weights, avoirdupois, 122-123
    volume, meaures of, 125
Tabulations, see Tables and charts
Tagliacozzo, Dr. Renata, 131-132
Tenses, 18-19
  in case reports, 31
  in description of observations, 31
  past, 31
  present, 31
  in summary of paper, 31
Terminations
  for gender of nouns, 103-104
  prescriptions, 128-130
Terminology, technical
  classical, 101-105
  confusion, 68
  excessive use of, 22-24
  foreign pharses and quotations, 67-69
  gobbledygook, 22-24
  illustration, 153
  usages, preferred, 65-67
Textbook material, 34-35

abbreviations, 108-117
  dates, 112
Theorists, 4
Time
  abbreviations, 114
  numbers, 119
  see also Weights, measures and time
Title, 36, 39-40
  ambiguity, 40
  English, 140-141
  foreign, 140-141
  in indexing, 40
  length, 39-40
  main, 39, 41-43
  misleading, 40
  subtitle, 39, 41-43
Title page, 135
Trademarked drugs, 127
  superior designation, 127
  see also, Pharmaceutic products and prescriptions
Trelease, S.F., and Yule, E.S., 178
Type, 45
  Greek letters and symbols, 45
  in illustrations, 149-154
  italics, 45
  labels, 151-154
  in preparation of manuscript, 144-148

U

UNESCO, United Nations Educational, Scientific and Cultural Organization, 68

V

Verbosity, 11-14
  deletions to improve, 11
  space takers or "running start," 12

W

Webster's New International Dictionary, 83, 86, 88
Weights, measures and time, 112-115
  abbreviations, 112-113
    in measurements, 112-115
    in ophthamology, 113
    in time, 114
  values, equivalent, 121-125

Index

equivalents, metric, 121-125
tables, *see* Individual heading
Who's Who, 86
Woglom, William H., 16, 46-47
Words and phrases, 46-82
  solecisms, 46-58
    abstract words in concrete sense, 50-51
    adjective modifying word other than one qualified, 55
    adjective as noun, 53-55
    biopsy, 58
    case, 49
    cystoscope, obstetricate, explore, refract, 53
    developed, 58
    dosage and dose, 51
    findings and found, 57-58
    group and type, 55-56
    histologic and histopathologic, 58
    indefinite article before name of condition, 56
    inject, 51-52
    medical jargon, 47-48
    milligrams per cent, 57
    operate, 56-57
    temperature and fever, and analogous expressions, 52-53
  usages, preferred, 65-67
    above and below, 64
    antepartum and prenatal, 80
    bilious, 64
    -derma, 81
    eczema, 64
    -emia words, 82
    epidemic encephalitis, 80
    eponym, 69-80
    foreign phrases, 67-69
      confusion of medical terms, 68
      stricter editing advised, 68-69
    gender of pronouns, 69
    infection *vs* infestation, 82
    infection *vs* inflammation, 65
    lymphogranuloma venerum, 81
    mongolians, mongoloids, 81
    neurasthenia, psychasthenia and hysteria, 64-65
    nomenclature of fungus diseases, 80
    nomenclature, official, 82
    phrases, overworked
    rheumatism, 65
    strain and sprain, 65
    superlatives, very, quite, marked, great, 62-63
  vague and inaccurate terms, 58-65
    ambiguous pronouns, 58-62
    multiple authors, 59-62
World Health Organization, 68
Writing
  fine or fancy, 8-11
    hyperbole, 11
    literary allusions, 9
    violations against, 11
  free-lance, viii

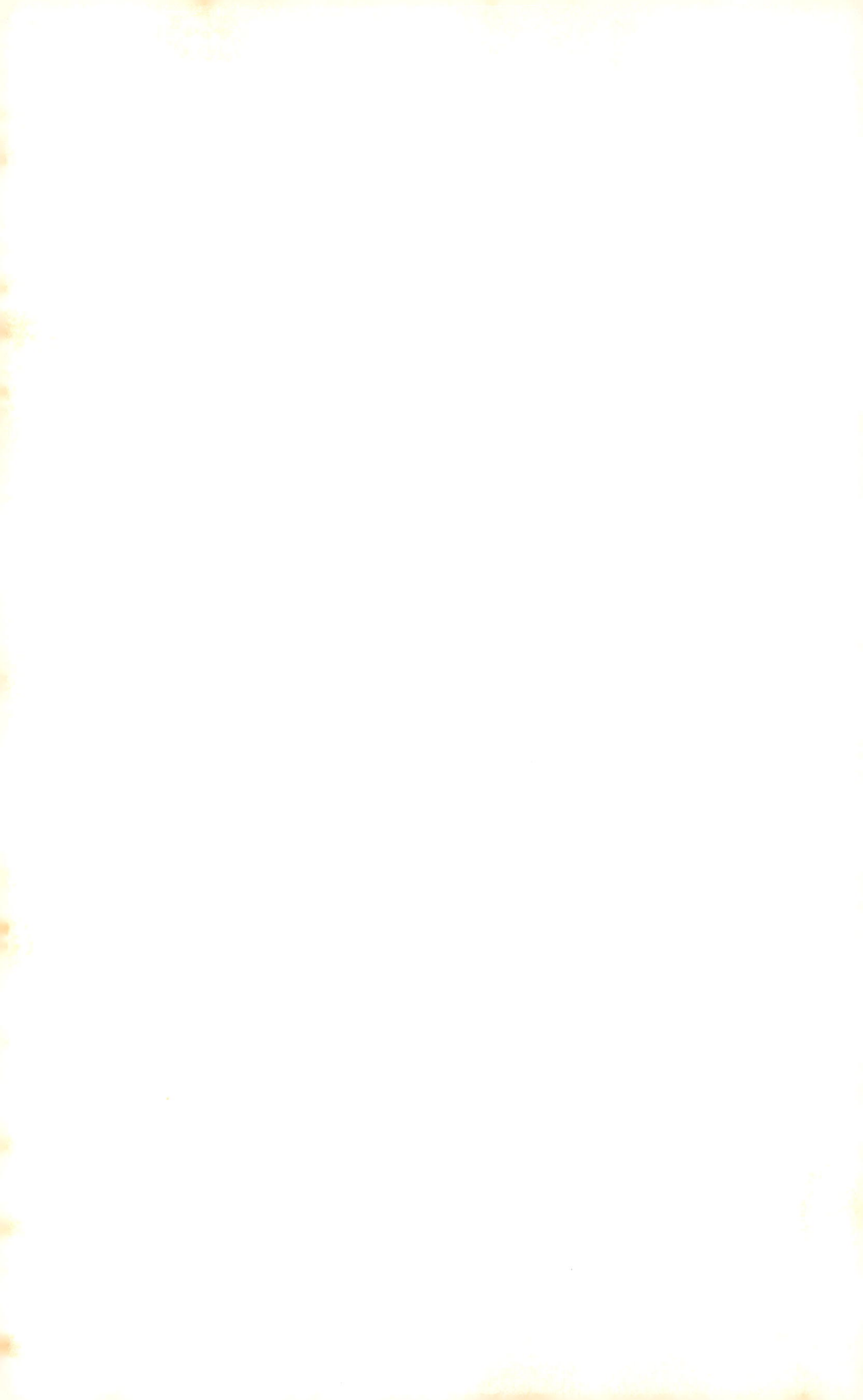